A Manual of
ELECTROTHERAPY

A Manual of
ELECTROTHERAPY

WILLIAM J. SHRIBER, M.A., M.D.

Assistant Professor of Medicine, Harvard Medical School;
Chief of Physical Medicine, Beth Israel Hospital;
Lecturer in Electrotherapy, Simmons College, Boston

FOURTH EDITION

LEA & FEBIGER

Philadelphia • *1975*

Library of Congress Cataloging in Publication Data

Shriber, William J.
  A manual of electrotherapy.

  First-3d ed. by A. L. Watkins.
  1. Electrotherapeutics. I. Watkins, Arthur Lancaster, 1909–   A manual
of electrotherapy. II. Title. [DNLM: 1. Electrotherapy. WB495 S56lm
1974]
RM871.S54   1974   615'.845   74-5307
ISBN 0-8121-0472-2

First Edition, 1958
Second Edition, 1962
Reprinted, 1965
Third Edition, 1968
Reprinted, 1970
Reprinted, 1972
Fourth Edition, 1975

Published in Great Britain by Henry Kimpton Publishers, London

Printed in the United States of America

Preface

This manual is an outgrowth of the book *Electrotherapy and Light Therapy*, first published in 1932 by Richard Kovacs "chiefly for physicians who were seeking unbiased guidance in the employment of electrotherapy and light therapy in their practice" and of a *Manual of Physical Therapy*, written by Dr. Kovacs for nurses. In 1958, Arthur Watkins, using both texts, presented *A Manual of Electrotherapy* for physical therapy students. It included the subjects of radiant energy, low-frequency and high-frequency currents, and ultrasound, since electricity was the apparent source of energy for each. Watkins also dealt with the methods of electrodiagnosis and electromyography.

Advances in medicine have brought about many changes in the clinical application of electrical apparatus. Diagnostic and therapeutic devices have been developed in answer to the demand. At one time, a variety of electrical stimulators were being developed for the treatment of muscle paralysis. The widespread prevention of paralytic poliomyelitis through immunization has altered not only the indications but also the instrumentation for electrical stimulation. Similarly, steroid and antibiotic drugs have changed the course and chronicity of disease, with subsequent alteration in the application of thermogenic agents.

In this fourth edition, the general arrangement of the subject matter has been retained. Additions and deletions throughout the book reflect the changing role of electrotherapy. Some forms of treatment have been discontinued in recent years; these methods are presented but are given less importance—e.g., the almost obsolete iontophoresis and galvanism.

Boston, Massachusetts   WILLIAM J. SHRIBER

Contents

PART I

Introduction

Chapter 1

SCOPE OF ELECTROTHERAPY

THE use of electrical energy in treatment, or electrotherapy, is an important part of physical therapy. It is necessary that the therapist be familiar with the elementary laws of electricity, as well as with the various modalities of treatment that have been developed over the years. The history of these developments makes interesting reading, but each new edition of this Manual deletes methods that are no longer generally used and concentrates only on the generally accepted and approved methods. Some reference is made to methods of treatment that are acceptable in some cities or states but not used in others.

The modality is selected by the physician writing the prescription. He may be a physiatrist (an accredited specialist in physical medicine) or any licensed physician, surgeon, or osteopath. If the physician is not familiar with the details of prescription writing, he may at times consult with the therapist about this important aspect of therapy. For this reason, some details of prescription writing will be discussed in this book.

Physical Therapy as Part of Practice of Medicine. One phase of physical therapy involves treating disease and injury with physical agents. As a rule, this kind of treatment is carried out in conjunction with medical and surgical measures, usually after a diagnosis has definitely been established. More is required of the therapist than turning on a switch. First, any measure to be applied must be based on a correct diagnosis and a definite conception of the existing pathological and functional changes. Information of this nature is provided by the physician. The second requirement is a knowledge of what the treatment is expected to accomplish; and third, there must be a full knowledge of just how that treatment is to be applied. Physical treatment must be as carefully prescribed and administered as any medicinal treatment, for it is axiomatic that any physical measure that is powerful enough to do good is capable of doing harm if incorrectly given. It is important, then, to know when to stop treatment. This decision is best made with the help of a specialist in physical medicine, or physiatrist.

Physical therapy rightfully forms part of the practice of medicine and surgery and is of most value in the treatment of disease and injury when employed by, or under the immediate supervision of, the physician who has learned why there is a scientific basis for the use of some physical energy or its combination with other measures, and who knows when and how to apply it.

Using electricity as the primary source of energy under discussion, let us consider some of the different methods used for therapeutic applications.

Radiant and Directly Applied Heat Methods. Heating devices are simplest and most commonly employed, both in the home and in the clinic. These include heating pads, usually thermostatically controlled, and radiant heat generators, typically incandescent lamps with some focusing shield provided, and, more recently, incandescent quartz rods giving off infrared light.

The primary effect in each instance is thermal; a secondary physiological effect is an increase in circulation. Some direct action on sensory nerves also may result, reducing pain. In any event, muscle spasm may be reduced, thus easing a painful area. The procedure or technique to be employed is selected by the physician writing the prescription.

Ultraviolet Radiation. Electric currents may be used to cause certain elements such as mercury, tungsten, or carbon to radiate energy in the invisible ultraviolet range of wavelengths. Such radiation produces photochemical effects in the skin (erythema) similar to sunburn. Its chief therapeutic use is in certain skin diseases. It is not of value for all types of rashes and may at times be dangerous in some diseases or in sensitive people. The secondary metabolic effects of ultraviolet are best known as they relate to the production of vitamin D in the body, but this is of little clinical significance today. The importance of exact prescription and dosage of ultraviolet radiation cannot be overemphasized (see Chapter 7).

Direct Current. This form of electrotherapy may be used for its effect on nerves and muscles causing muscular contractions and in electrodiagnosis. Direct currents have been popular in the past because of their polar effects on ionized molecules, causing them to be driven through the skin, usually superficially. This is known as iontophoresis or ion transfer.

Direct currents also have some counterirritant action on the skin and may cause local vasodilation. Because they stimulate sensory nerve endings, they cause pleasant or painful effects, dependent on dosage.

The direct current is also used in electrodiagnosis and to measure skin resistance.

Repetitive (Low-Frequency) Currents. Stimulation of nerves and muscles by repetitive currents of proper frequency and intensity will cause sustained contraction in muscles. This action of electrical stimulation on muscles is used clinically as an aid in muscle re-education; for passive exercise when the lower motor neuron is intact; for passive exercise in lower motor neuron disease; and occasionally in hysterical paralysis. These currents are essential in electrodiagnostic studies. Their use in electroshock therapy and in cardiac stimulation is not included in this text. A most recent method of application is surface electrical stimulation for suppression of intractable pain.

High-Frequency Currents. Electrical currents of frequency greater than a million cycles per second (cps) heat tissues when properly applied. This method of heating is called short-wave diathermy. Extremely high-frequency currents with shorter wavelengths are called microwaves and constitute another method of deep heating electrically. These methods are discussed in later chapters.

Ultrasound. High-frequency currents in the neighborhood of a million cycles per second may be used to generate vibratory or sound energy. This energy has a deep-heating effect often called diathermy and is included as a part of electrotherapy.

The student of physical therapy must understand that any form of physical energy applied to the body first exerts a physical action known as the "primary" physical effect which in turn brings on "secondary" physiological effects. The influence on organic or functional changes in the body will, therefore, be in direct relation to the extent of the primary physical changes. Hence, the necessity of a careful technique and measured dosage in the application of all physical agents.

Most of the procedures and effects of physical measures are applied through the skin. The skin is not merely a protective covering of the body but is also a complex structure capable of perception, absorption, and excretion. It is capable of a variety of reactions to stimuli from the outside and from within. Most of the reactions brought about by physical forces are nonspecific in character. It has been shown that stimuli of different nature, such as heat, manipulation, and chemical or electrical agents, cause similar vascular response in the skin, consisting of dilatation of blood vessels, increased permeability of the vessel wall, and increased circulation. The nervous reflex effect upon deeper parts may be alike in every instance, and this explains the paradox of the similar therapeutic effects of physical agents of apparently different nature. There are, on the other hand, specific skin reactions that can be produced by only one agent, such as those caused by ultraviolet radiation. With physical agents capable of penetrating the protective covering of the skin and other tissues, specific effects on inner organs can be expected. This part of physical therapy is still a fertile field for clinical research.

Simple Measures vs. Apparatus It is by no means necessary to possess a large array of machinery to produce the few basic physical and physiological effects: Simple hot and cold applications and active and passive exercise can do a world of good by themselves. There is danger in too much and too complicated apparatus for physical therapy, just as there is danger of too much apparatus for diagnostic purposes when one's five senses and clinical experience, unaided, should be adequate to solve many problems. On the other hand, modern mechanical and electrical progress offers many types of efficient apparatus that conserves one's own body energy and saves time in accomplishing results. The advantages of modern electrical and light apparatus over some of the older devices are just as evident as those of the modern methods of transportation over the time-honored mode of walking and pushcarts. The finer and more varied the control and the more accurate the measurement of energy output, the more efficient and the more dependable will be the subsequent physiological and clinical results.

Classification. The classification of physical therapy methods for instruction purposes presents a somewhat involved problem. It would seem logical to group together physical measures that have the same physiological effect, just as in medicinal therapy drugs of the same effect are presented in one group. Such grouping, however, would lead to some confusion and repetition and is not suitable for didactic purposes. For the purposes of this manual, however, certain aspects of thermotherapy, light therapy, electrodiagnosis, electrotherapy, diathermy, and ultrasound will be considered. As the primary source of energy in each instance is electricity, the general term electrotherapy is employed.

Chapter 2

HISTORY OF ELECTROTHERAPY

THE shocks of the torpedo, an electric fish, were prescribed by Ætius, a Greek physician, for the treatment of gout. Paracelsus, the leading medical man of the Middle Ages, believed that the magnet had power over all diseases. The book of William Gilbert, physician to Queen Elizabeth, published in 1600, *De Magnete,* was the first to awaken interest in the use of electricity for treatment. Gilbert discovered that glass, sulfur, resin, and many other substances shared the capacity of amber to attract light objects when rubbed. He coined the name "electricity" (electricitas) from the Greek word "electron" for amber. In 1780, Galvani, professor of anatomy at the University of Bologna, first observed the twitching of muscles under the influence of electricity in a nerve-muscle preparation of a frog's leg. Seeking the cause of this, the idea of animal electricity came to him. Galvani then proved that atmospheric electricity as manifested in lightning would produce the same effects on muscular movements. He placed an atmospheric conductor on the highest point of his house and from this he ran down a wire to his laboratory and attached it to a frog leg preparation; whenever lightning flashed from the clouds, the limbs of the animals underwent violent contractions. Next, another Italian, Alessandro Volta, professor of natural philosophy, proved that electricity in Galvani's experiments was not inherent in the animal, but was due to a flow of current between two dissimilar metals when they are placed in contact. In the spring of 1800, he made a pile of metal discs of zinc and copper, placing moist cloth instead of a frog's muscles between them; from here it was an easy step to placing the two metals in a vessel filled with acidulated water. This was the invention of the electric cell or battery.

Functional machines and the galvanic battery served as the early sources of energy for electrotherapy. The discovery of the Leyden jar in 1745 enabled the storing up of a powerful charge of electricity; with the shocks from this jar, the famous Abbé Nollet administered, in the presence of the King of France, a shock to 180 of the royal guard simultaneously.

The first book on electrotherapy was published in 1745 by a German physician, Kratzenstein. His method of treatment consisted of seating

7

the patient on a wooden stool, electrifying him by means of a large re-volving frictional glass globe and then drawing sparks from him. Kratzen-stein explained his results by the driving out of excess blood from the affected tissues. [7]Jallabert, of Paris, first advocated the use of electric sparks for muscular contractions, and[8] Marat, the revolutionist, wrote a book on the treatment of paralysis, hemiplegia, rheumatism and other conditions by electricity. He insisted that the duration of treatment should be definitely fixed and that there should be a dosage of electricity as well as of medicines.[9] John Wesley, the great divine, published a book on electrical treatment in 1780. The first hospital physical therapy de-partment ever organized was the electrical department at Guy's Hospital in London under Dr.[10] Golding Bird in 1840.

Following the epoch-making discovery of the induction coil by[11] Fara-day, the laws of electrophysiology, or stimulation of muscles and nerves by the galvanic and faradic current, were developed in the middle of the last century by Du[14] Bois-Reymond and[15] Duchenne of France and[16] Erb of Germany. [12]John H. Kellogg, of Battle Creek, Michigan, described in 1888 the use of the sinusoidal current for muscle stimulation.[18] Tesla's discovery of high-frequency currents led[19] d'Arsonval in 1892 to experiment with their use in treatment. Diathermy was described in the first decade of this century by[20] Zeynek and Nagelschnidt of Germany and was further[21] developed by F.[22] deKraft of New York for medical uses and by[23] Clark of Philadelphia for surgery. Short-wave diathermy was developed by [24]Schereschewsky and Whitney[25] of the United States and by Schliephake[26] of Germany. Microwave diathermy originated from wartime radar, based on the construction of the magnetron tube by Sir[27] Arthur Tisdale of Eng-land. A reversion to the earlier methods of treatment by electric shock has occurred in recent years, with low-frequency alternating currents ad-ministered to the brain for treatment of depressive mental conditions.

ADDITIONAL READING

Licht, S. H.: History of electrotherapy, pp. 1–69. In S. Licht (ed.), *Therapeutic Electricity and Ultraviolet Radiation*. 2nd ed. Licht, New Haven, Conn., 1967.

PART II

Heat Energy

Chapter 3

PHYSICS AND PHYSIOLOGICAL
EFFECTS OF HEAT

Physics of Heat. Heat is the term used to describe the energy that matter can store in the form of electronic, atomic, or molecular vibrations. Higher heat energy means higher temperatures.

Cold in a physical sense is a negative condition, depending on the decrease in the amount of molecular vibration that constitutes heat. We speak of bodies as hot or cold, according to the way in which they affect our temperature sense. When a hot body is brought into contact with a cold body, the former is cooled while the latter is warmed. The exchange of heat between two bodies that are at different temperature results in a gain of heat to the colder body and a net loss of heat from the hotter body until they finally arrive at the same temperature. Temperature plays, therefore, the same part in the flow of heat as pressure does in the flow of water: Heat always passes from the hot to the cooler body. If the human body is brought close to a cooler object, the latter will abstract heat from the body and give rise to the *sensation* of cold.

According to the kinetic theory of heat, temperature is a measure of the average amount of kinetic energy possessed by each individual molecule of a body. The intensity of heat in a body is measured by the temperature. For purposes of human biology, temperatures may be classified as follows:

Very cold	32° to 55° F
Cold	55° to 65° F
Cool	65° to 80° F
Neutral	80° to 92° F
Warm	92° to 98° F.
Hot	98° to 104° F
Very hot	104° F and above

Sources of Heat. The three principal sources of heat are chemical action, electric currents, and mechanical work, including friction.

Production of heat by *chemical action* is exemplified by the burning or oxidation of wood, gas, oil, and coal; another example is the adding of cold water to lime, which brings about an instantaneous production of heat. Chemical reactions in the body or body metabolism produce heat and maintain body temperature. An *electric current* moving against electric resistance produces heat. All conductors of electricity convert part or all of the electrical energy flowing through them into heat energy. Electric heaters, toasters, irons, and incandescent lamps operate on this principle. Similarly, a high-frequency current generates heat as a result of the resistance of tissues to the passage of high-frequency current. *Mechanical action* in the form of friction, compression, or percussion converts the kinetic energy of a moving mass gradually or suddenly into heat energy. Parts of machinery rubbing against each other create heat. Massage of a friction type can increase skin temperature. The newest method of producing heat from mechanical energy is the application of ultrasonic vibrations.

Transmission of Heat. Heat energy may be transferred from one place to another by three processes: conduction, convection, and radiation. 4. Conversion - from one form to another form of energy.

1 In *conduction*, transfer of heat energy from a hot body to a cold one takes place in and through matter by molecular collision. If one end of a metal spoon is held in a flame, the other end soon becomes unbearably hot. Good conductors of heat like metals are generally good conductors of electricity.

2 In *convection*, heat transference takes place by movements of a mass. When rooms are heated by a hot stove, the air in contact with the stove becomes warm, expands, and is pushed up by the cooler heavier air. Liquids and gases are heated principally by convection.

3 In *radiation*, the objects between which transference of heat occurs are separated by an intervening medium that does not itself become warmed by the heat transmitted through it. The earth is warmed by its chief source of heating, the sun's radiation, without the warming of the intervening atmosphere. Heating of a body by the radiation from the sun or from a fire occurs by absorption of the radiant energy.

In addition, heat energy may be generated by conversion from some other form of energy. High-frequency electrical currents (diathermy) or high-frequency mechanical energy (ultrasound) can penetrate the skin and soft tissues; the absorbed energy is converted to heat, causing deep local temperature changes.

Forms of Therapeutic Heating. Heating for treatment purposes may be derived from numerous sources, as shown in Table 3–1. These may be classified under three main headings:

1. *Conductive and Convective Sources.* Hot-water bottles, poultices, and fomentations are popular home devices for local heating, but they are not efficient, because their source of heating is not constant, their heat penetration is limited, and, furthermore, they are cumbersome and often unbearable on account of the pressure exerted. Electric heating pads are more convenient because they are of light weight and their temperature

Table 3–1.   Sources of Therapeutic Heating

Source	Form of Energy	Heat Transmitted
Hot-water bottle Hot moist pack Hot-water bath Paraffin bath Electric heating pad	Molecular motion	By conduction and convection
Infrared radiator (non-luminous)	Long-wave infrared rays	By radiation
Heat lamp (incandescent bulb) and (incandescent) quartz rod Sun	Short-wave infrared rays, visible rays Infrared, visible and ultraviolet rays	By radiation
Short-wave diathermy Microwave diathermy Ultrasound	High-frequency electrical oscillations High-frequency mechanical oscillation	By conversion of oscillations

can be evenly maintained and also adjusted at two or three levels by suitable resistance units. Well-constructed electric blankets serve for making beds warm and for keeping patients at constant comfortable warmth.

Other conductive sources for efficient local heating are the paraffin bath, which produces high surface heating as well as heat retention in the depth; and the whirlpool bath, which offers a combination of heat and mild friction and enables exercise of the immersed parts. Hot-water baths are convenient sources for heating the skin and superficial tissues, but their penetrating effect is very limited; with surface temperatures that can be safely tolerated, the deep-lying tissues dissipate heat through the vascular bed at a faster rate than it can be conducted to them.

2. *Radiant Sources.* Heat lamps and infrared heating units have come into general use on account of simplicity and safety of application. Their rays penetrate the superficial layers of the skin. The heat energy is then conducted slowly to the deeper layers. The luminous quartz rod, called a "Z-500" Infrared Lamp by the Burdick Corp., has an output in the near infrared zone that permits good penetration and hence heating effect.

3. *Conversive Sources.* Diathermy, or the passage of a high-frequency current through a part, results in its conversion into heat. Diathermy enables penetrating tissue heating and the treatment of deeper parts. It will be discussed in Chapter 16.

Ultrasound application allows a type of high-frequency mechanical energy (vibrations) to enter deep tissues, where it is converted into heat. This subject will be discussed in Chapter 17.

Physical Effects of Heating. No matter what form of heating is applied to the body, its immediate effect is purely physical: a rise of temperature in the tissues to which heat is directed. The degree and extent of this primary heat effect will vary according to the source of heating, its intensity, and the length of application. The heat tolerance of the parts also plays a role. For treatment purposes, no form of heating should ever be applied beyond the limits of comfortable toleration. The average maximum tolerance of the skin to radiant heating has been shown to be 113.9° F for the surface and 117.8° for the undersurface. Tests of the uterus indicate some rise of temperature of inner organs produced by diathermy. General body temperature can be elevated to 107° F by artificial hyperpyrexia for short periods.

According to the temperature law of Van't Hoff, for every rise of 10° C the rate of oxidation is increased 2.5 times, and thus temperature changes of even tenths of degrees will influence cellular oxidations and exert marked effects on physiological processes.

Physical losses of heat during thermal applications should be considered. These may occur by reflection, convection, and radiation. Radiant heat is reflected especially by shiny white surfaces; reflection is not much of a factor in human skin. Convective heat losses may be important. For this reason, skin areas exposed to radiant heat sources should be protected against drafts. All objects radiate heat, including the human body. To prevent heat loss by radiation, the exposed skin should not be near a large object or surface that is at a lower temperature.

Physiological Effects of Heating. The heat-regulating mechanism of the body maintains a constant temperature. When heat is applied to a part from an external source, the vasomotor mechanism responds in an effort to dissipate the excess heat by active vasodilatation of the capillaries and by an increase of arterial and venous circulation. Lewis has shown that irritation of the tissues releases a histaminelike substance that causes dilatation of the capillaries. The local hyperemia in turn results in an increase of the rate of removal of local tissue products and in stimulation of the local resistive forces, such as increased phagocytosis and lymph flow.

Local heating in mild dosage acts as a sedative on irritative conditions of sensory and motor nerves. This explains the relief given by thermal measures in many painful sensory conditions and in cramps and spasm. Often heat may be more effective in reducing pain than strong narcotic drugs.

When heat is applied at sufficient intensity to a large part of the body or when the normal heat loss from the body is prevented, a rise of body temperature and general physiological changes occur. There is an increase of the circulatory rate and of metabolism, a rise in blood volume and oxygen consumption, and a change in the urine, blood, and sweat to the alkaline side.

The clinical effects of mild general body heating can be summed up as follows: (1) increased heat elimination and profuse perspiration; (2) increased circulation, a rise of the pulse rate in the ratio of about 10 beats for every degree Fahrenheit, just as in fever; (3) a lowering of blood pressure (in contrast to the effects of cold); (4) increased respiration; (5) increased elimination through the kidneys. There is a loss of water, salt, and urea and other nitrogenous substances, with a relative excess of alkali remaining in the blood and in the tissues, while there is also a temporary loss of body weight. General nervous sensibility is usually markedly lessened. The enumerated physiological effects of local and general heating are the basis of the extensive clinical use of the diverse forms of heating.

ADDITIONAL READING

Brengelmann, G. L.: Temperature regulation, pp. 105–135. In T. C. Ruch and H. D. Patton (eds.), *Physiology and Biophysics, Vol. III: Digestion, Metabolism, Endocrine Function and Reproduction.* 20th ed. W. B. Saunders, Philadelphia, 1973.

Downey, J. A., and Darling, R. C.: Special review: Thermotherapy and thermoregulation. Amer. J. Phys. Med., 43:265, 1964.

Fischer, E., and Soloman, S.: Physiological responses to heat and cold, pp. 126–169. In S. Licht (ed.), *Therapeutic Heat and Cold.* 2nd ed. Waverly Press, Baltimore, 1965.

Hardy, J. D.: Physiology of temperature regulation. Physiol. Rev., 41:521, 1961.

Lewis, T.: *The Blood Vessels of the Human Skin and Their Responses.* Shaw and Sons, London, 1927.

Chapter 4

PHYSICS OF RADIANT ENERGY

General Considerations. We are now to present the therapeutic aspects of a broad division of physical science, that of radiant energy. Radiation is the process by which energy may be propagated through empty space. Every substance with a temperature above absolute zero emits radiant energy in the form of heat radiation. When electrical or chemical forces of suitable intensity are applied to various forms of matter, luminous and other forms of radiations may be produced. Infrared, visible, and ultraviolet rays all are forms of radiant energy. The common characteristics of all forms of radiant energy are as follows: they are produced by applying electrical and other forces to various forms of matter; they all may be transmitted without the support of a sensible medium; their velocity of travel is equal in vacuum but varies in different media. Their direction of propagation is normally a straight line; they undergo reflection, deflection, and absorption by media. They are designated collectively as electromagnetic radiations. All such radiations consist of a train of electromagnetic oscillations moving as a sequence of waves. The various radiations differ only in their wavelengths, i.e., in the spacing between successive wave crests.

Light is a form of radiant energy that makes objects visible by stimulating the retina of the eye. Ultraviolet and infrared radiation do not render objects visible. The general terms light therapy and phototherapy by custom include the employment of the visible as well as invisible radiations of heat and ultraviolet or actinic rays, because they are all, as a rule, produced at the same time and the therapeutic results are due to their combined effect. The term actinotherapy relates more specifically to the employment of ultraviolet radiation.

The application of radiant energy for the treatment of disease or the stimulation of lagging biological processes forms one of the most interesting and most complex chapters of present-day physical therapy. A maze of clinical and experimental material has been accumulated in recent years on every phase of the subject. For the purpose of this volume, only the basic physical and physiological facts and the practical uses of infrared, visible, and ultraviolet radiation will be presented. Roentgen rays and radioactivity, although in a physical sense part of radiant energy, are not included in this consideration because, by well-established custom, they form part of another large special field of the practice of medicine·

Classification of Radiant Energy. If a beam of white light passes through a glass prism, it is not only refracted but also dispersed, and a series of colored bands called a spectrum is seen in the prism (Fig. 4–1). Each color corresponds to a different kind of radiation, and their appearance is due to the fact that each is refracted differently. The radiation producing the sensation of red is refracted least, and that producing the sensation of violet is refracted most. Beyond the part of the spectrum that affects the retina, the visible rays, there are invisible rays. A thermometer or thermocouple placed beyond the red side of the visible spectrum will register heat, and a sensitive photographic plate held beyond the violet will register chemical changes. The longer-wavelength rays beyond the red end are called infrared, and the shorter-wavelength rays beyond the violet end are known as ultraviolet rays. It has been found that the visible spectrum comprises only a small part of the full range of radiant energy. At the red end there exists a large region of radiations designated as infrared, and next to these another very large range of radiations that are the so-called radio or Hertzian waves. At the violet end of the visible spectrum, there is the region of ultraviolet rays, and beyond these are the roentgen rays and the gamma rays.

The graphic representation of the various energy waves as a function of wavelength is known as the *electromagnetic spectrum.* The basis of comparison of the different parts of the electromagnetic spectrum, besides their physical and physiological effects, is either their wavelength (the distance between the crests of two successive waves) or their frequency of vibration. Since all electromagnetic energy travels at the same velocity through vacuum and air, it is evident that the shorter waves must vibrate at a greater frequency and *vice versa.* A homely comparison to visualize this may be a motley army of giants and dwarfs, all under orders to reach the same goal simultaneously; in order to do so the giants step out leisurely, while the dwarfs run and take hundreds of steps for

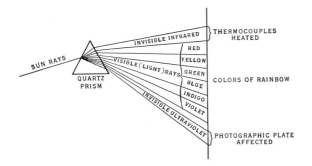

Fig. 4–1.   Component parts of solar radiation.

each one of the giants. Dividing 186,000 miles (or 3×10^8 meters) per second, the uniform speed of radiant energy in vacuum, by the wavelength furnishes the wave frequency or the rate of passage of wave crests per second. One can classify electromagnetic radiations either by their wavelength or by their frequency, as is done with the radio waves. The frequencies of the different forms of electromagnetic radiation used in therapy are so very great that it would be impracticable to use such huge figures. The classification of the therapeutic parts of the electromagnetic spectrum is, therefore, made by stating their wavelengths.

Table 4–1 shows the subdivision, physical characteristics, sources, and therapeutic classification of the entire range of electromagnetic radiations.

Unit of Wavelength. The metric system is used to designate wavelength. For radiant energy used therapeutically—namely, infrared, visible and ultraviolet rays—the wavelengths are extremely short, so that one speaks in terms of millimicrons ($m\mu$), or one millionth of a millimeter (mm). The angstrom unit (Å), found in the earlier literature, is one tenth of a millimicron. At the present time, wavelength is more frequently measured in millimicrons ($m\mu$) or nanometers (nm): 1 nm is equal to 1 $m\mu$. (See Table 4–2.)

Table 4–1. The Electromagnetic Spectrum

Discoverer	Date	Wavelength (in Air) millimicrons	Designation	Frequency per Second	Medical Use
Millikan	1921	0.0001	cosmic	3×10^{21}	not known
The Curies Becquerel	1898	0.01	gamma	3×10^{18}	radium therapy
Roentgen	1895	50	x ray	5.9×10^{15}	diagnosis and therapy
Ritter	1801	300	ultraviolet	7.5×10^{14}	diagnosis, vitamin D, germicidal and therapy
Newton	1704	400–800	visible	3.7×10^{14}	not known
		millimeters			
Herschel	1839	0.001–0.1	infrared	3×10^{11}	superficial tissue radiant heating
Hertz	1886	0.5–100	microwave	1×10^{10}	diathermy heating
		meters			
Maxwell	1865	10–30	short-wave	3×10^6	diathermy heating, surgical diathermy
		10–30	television		
		300	radio	3×10^4	audiomental stimulation
Faraday	1831	5×10^{10}	electric power	60	electrotherapy, neural and muscular stimulation

Theory of Radiant Energy. For many years, the commonly accepted theory of radiant energy was that electromagnetic radiations gave rise to waves of the ether, the theoretical substance which was supposed to be an unbroken entity throughout the universe. This is known as Maxwell's electromagnetic theory, dating back to its announcement by that brilliant physicist, in 1868, when it replaced the old "corpuscular" theory of Newton. Newer investigations have led to a modified return of the old Newtonian conception of light as a definite entity.

According to our present knowledge, a light ray consists of an enormously large number of exceedingly small entities known as photons. In a sense they are the indivisible units of radiant energy. Photons are produced by high-velocity electronic or molecular motion or by release of kinetic energy through collision of molecules. In gas and vapor discharges such as the mercury or neon lamps, photons are produced by the energy released when a displaced electron regains a normal orbital position about an ion or atom. The photon is ejected from a light source at a velocity of 186,000 miles per second in vacuum, a speed it maintains until slowed or stopped by a medium such as a liquid or solid body. Photons exert a pressure upon any object that they strike, for they possess inertia. Thus they appear to be material particles, but while in flight they exhibit many properties associated with wave forms of energy. This kind of radiation, whether roentgen ray, ultraviolet, or infrared, exhibits wavelike characteristics in certain phenomena; in other instances, it behaves like bullets shot from a gun except that these bullets are just as potent at 100 yards as at 1 yard. The energy content of each photon is determined by the frequency of vibration of the wave.

The amount of energy carried by a particular photon is proportional to the frequency. Since wavelength varies inversely with frequency, a photon at 200 mμ will have twice the energy content of a photon at 400 mμ. This is one reason roentgen rays, which have very small wavelengths, of the order of 1.0 mμ, have much greater destructive power on tissue

Table 4–2. Wavelengths of Radiations

Radiation	Wavelength
Very long electric waves	5,000,000 m
Radio waves	30,000 to 1 m
Commercial broadcast	600 to 200 m
Amateur broadcast	175 to 20 m
International broadcast	50 to 15 m
High-frequency (long-wave diathermy)	300 m
High-frequency (short-wave diathermy)	30 to 3 m
Microwave	0.5 to 100 cm
Infrared rays	100,000 to 770 mμ
Visible rays	770 to 390 mμ
Ultraviolet rays	390 to 13.6 mμ
Roentgen rays	13.6 to 0.14 mμ
Gamma rays	0.14 to 0.001 mμ

than ultraviolet radiations. Infrared radiations have lower radiation frequency and longer wavelengths than ultraviolet, so that the lower-energy
photons serve chiefly to increase the kinetic or thermal energy of the
molecules in the absorbing media.

Measuring Radiant Energy. In checking the efficiency of his sources
of radiation, the average physician can employ simple clinical tests, as
described for ultraviolet radiation (p. 61), which merely indicate the presence and the gross intensity of certain wavelengths—those causing dermatitis or sunburn. For accurate measurements, he will have to depend on the
laboratory services furnished by the manufacturer of his lamp or by an
independent physicist. For this purpose, chemical as well as photoelectric methods have been developed by some investigators; the basic method appears to be the radiometric one. Its principle is the use of a thermopile connected with a high-sensitivity galvanometer. These radiometers
are equally sensitive to all wavelengths of the radiant energy spectrum.
All energy, regardless of wavelength, is transformed into heat when absorbed by the receiving area of the instrument; the intensity is expressed
quantitatively as the number of calories, joules, or ergs of heat produced
per unit of area of absorbing surface per second. The interposition of
suitably calibrated filters, which in turn absorb either the infrared or
luminous or ultraviolet energy, makes it possible to obtain the percentages
of these radiations present in the total radiation exposure. Comparison
with previous calibration against a radiation standard makes it possible
to specify the intensity of the energy incident at the point where measurement is made, in gram calories per square centimeter per second or watts
per cm^2.

Spectroscopic Comparison. The term spectrogram denotes a charted
band of wavelengths of electromagnetic radiation obtained by refraction
or diffraction by means of a prism or grating. For determining the wavelength variation of the transmission of substances in the ultraviolet and
visible regions, spectrograms are all that are necessary. Spectra can be
classified into three kinds: (1) Continuous spectra are those emitted by
incandescent solid substances, such as the sun, the carbon arc lamp, and
incandescent lamps; they are pure thermal radiations and contain a continuous scale of wavelengths, the extent and energy distribution of which
depend on the temperature of the hot body. (2) Line spectra are emitted
by incandescent vapors and gases, such as mercury vapor; they consist of
more or less sharply defined lines that are generally distributed without
any apparent regularity. No two elements give spectral lines in exactly
the same position in the spectrogram and thus an element may be detected merely by observing its spectral lines. The present view is that
these lines are produced by the "falling in" of electrons that have been
displaced from their normal orbits or "shells." (3) Banded spectra are
given by compounds when these are dissociated; they always can be re-
solved into groups of fine lines.

Comparative spectrograms of the various sources of light are of little value in judging the amount of energy produced by the light source. It has been stated that, on the basis of a spectrogram, the ideal ultraviolet source would be the automobile spark plug operated on the automobile ignition system, for it gives a better spectrogram than can be obtained by the quartz mercury arc or any of the carbon arcs. Spectrograms must, therefore, be completed by a chart or table showing the light energy present at each wavelength. In comparing the graphic representation of energy distribution from various sources at different wavelengths, the strength of the activating current must also be stated, for it makes a difference if one set of curves is produced by a 30-ampere source and the other by a 5-ampere source. Comparative spectrograms are of value only if taken under identical conditions of distance, energy input, and exposure time and on plates of equal sensitivity.

Common Physical Phenomena. The following physical phenomena may occur when electromagnetic radiations encounter other substances:

1. The rays are reflected or thrown back. Snow is an excellent reflector of ultraviolet energy. The reflectors mounted around the various lamps reflect both visible and invisible radiations and add to its amount. When skin scales are present, they reflect a certain amount of radiation, and the length of exposure has to be somewhat increased.

2. The rays penetrate. Clear liquids, glass, and quartz are more transparent to light rays than to heat rays. The various layers of the skin and various glasses are variously transparent to certain wavelengths (Fig. 4–2). The rays are refracted when a beam of light passes obliquely from one medium to another: The rays are bent at the surface separating the two media.

3. The rays are absorbed. Secondary to this absorption, chemical and biological phenomena result, such as fluorescence, phosphorescence, ionization, photoelectric effect, and chemical catalysis. The discussion of these purely photophysical effects is beyond the scope of this presentation.

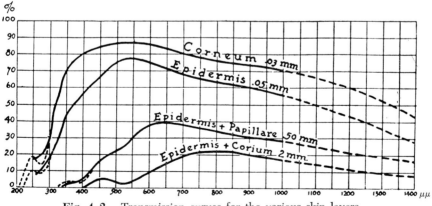

Fig. 4–2. Transmission curves for the various skin layers.

The Inverse Square Law. It is a fact that the intensity of radiation varies inversely with the square of the distance from the source. This would imply that technicians must not decrease the distance of a lamp from the body without careful calculation, in order to prevent overexposure. However, this law applies only to point sources or sources at such a distance from the observer that they approximate a compact source. The law cannot be applied to lamps that have reflectors, nor is it valid if reflections from walls and ceilings are substantial.

The Angulation of Rays (Cosine Law). Patients receive optimum radiation if the source of radiation is at right angles to the center of the area to be radiated. For instance, at two-thirds of a right angle (30 degrees) double exposure is necessary to produce the same intensity as at 90 degrees. With deviation less than 30 degrees, the small loss of radiation can be disregarded.

Chapter 5

INFRARED AND LUMINOUS RADIATION

Physical Considerations. Any object heated to a higher temperature than its surroundings will send out its excess of heat by radiation to the surrounding objects. An iron rod when heated first "feels" hot without showing any change in color (so-called black-body radiation), then starts glowing and becomes "red hot" and later "white-hot." At each stage of heating, a variety of radiation is emitted; in the stage of low heat there is long-wave or far-infrared radiation, invisible to the eye; at a further stage of heat, the red, green and blue rays of the visible spectrum are added, and at the stage of white heat the presence of ultraviolet radiation can be demonstrated. The quality as well as the quantity of radiations emitted from any source depends not only on the physical properties of the source itself but also on the energy input, which governs the intensity of heat generated in the radiating object: the hotter the source, the shorter the wavelength.

The generally accepted classification differentiates between two groups of infrared radiations:

Long-Wave Infrared. These rays are emitted by all heated bodies, and exclusively by low-temperature bodies such as hot-water bottles, electric heating pads, and dull red heaters. Their wavelengths extend mostly from 1,500 to 12,000 millimicrons; they do not penetrate tissue deeper than 2 millimeters and are strongly absorbed in the upper layers of skin (upper 0.5 mm).

Short-Wave Infrared. These rays are emitted by all incandescent bodies such as the sun, electric arc, incandescent lamps, and specially designed high-temperature infrared radiators. They comprise radiations between 700 and 1,500 millimicrons in wavelength. The employment of a special red glass filter restricts these sources to such wavelengths exclusively. They can penetrate through 5 to 10 mm of skin tissue. They are, therefore, able to influence blood vessels, lymph vessels, nerve endings and other subcutaneous tissue directly.

SOURCES OF INFRARED RADIATION

Sunlight is the most important natural source of infrared radiation: Infrared radiation comprises over 60 per cent of the radiation in average sunlight, the rest being mainly ultraviolet and visible light. In everyday practice, various types of infrared generators are the most convenient and most popular sources of external heating.

Artificial sources of infrared are divided into two groups: low-temperature or nonluminous sources or infrared radiators and high-temperature or luminous sources or heat lamps. As a matter of fact, in both groups infrared radiation is the chief heating factor. In both groups, the means for generating heat are metallic conductors that become heated by the passage of an electric current. For low-temperature heating, a bare wire or carbon held in suitable nonconducting material is employed; for high-temperature heating, the oxidation of the wire must be prevented, and hence the use of tungsten enclosed in an evacuated or inert-gas-filled glass bulb. High-temperature generators emit a large amount of luminous radiation. In actual practice, the so-called nonluminous sources always attain a red glow and emit a quantity of visible red radiation; hence, their designation as nonluminous is not entirely correct.

Heat Lamps. Heat lamps or incandescent filament radiators are the principal sources of luminous heat radiation. They consist of tungsten filaments enclosed in a glass bulb mounted at the center of a concave reflector. These lamps come in different sizes, varying from 150 to 1500 watts.

The penetration of the radiation from these luminous heat generators through the skin is the same whether they are of small (150 to 250 watts) or large (1500) wattage. The principal difference in the use of the smaller and larger lamps is that the former serve for treatment of small areas, such as the face, shoulders, hands, or feet, while the large lamps can warm up larger areas of the body, such as the entire back or abdomen or both legs (Figs. 5–1 and 5–2).

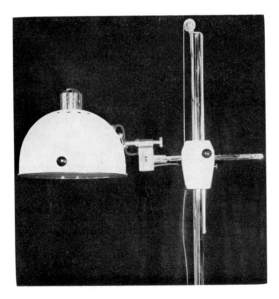

Fig. 5–1. Large luminous heat lamp on stand.

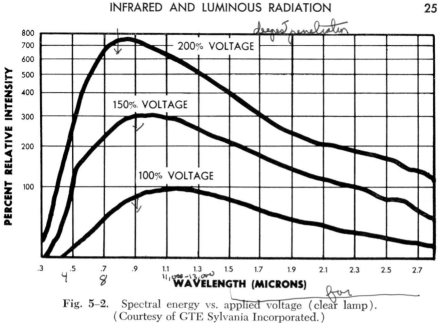

Fig. 5–2.   Spectral energy vs. applied voltage (clear lamp).
(Courtesy of GTE Sylvania Incorporated.)

Two or more incandescent bulbs of low power (25 to 60 watts) mounted in semicircular containers are designated as electric light "bakers." The term originated from the resemblance of this heating device to an oven. In contrast to the high temperatures needed for real "baking," resulting in the coagulation of albumen, the temperature rise in the skin produced by these bakers never exceeds more than about 110° F under safe limits. Heat lamps mounted on stands are more easily moved about than some of the older heavy bakers.

An improved and inexpensive newer source of short-wave infrared as well as visible radiation is a tungsten filament in a conical gas-filled glass bulb, which screws into any electric lamp socket. These are often made with Pyrex to eliminate breakage.

Quartz Infrared Lamp.   This source of heat is similar to a quartz broiler for cooking. The electrical energy is ordinary 115-volt house current. The lamp consists of a tungsten filament sealed in a gas-filled quartz tube or bulb. The lamps operate at a very high radiating efficiency, and the filament heats up or cools down in less than a second (Fig. 5–8).

Infrared nonluminous generators consist of a heating element that is mounted in the center of a parabolic reflector and warmed by an electrical current to a dull red heat. The reflector should concentrate the heat rays on the surface of the body, evenly and without hot spots. In the popularly known bathroom heater, which is also an infrared generator, the wide hood reflects the rays over a wide area, and the heater itself is not adjustable. The heating element consists of either a resistance wire wound around or embedded in a nonconducting material (porcelain or steatite) or a rod or circular plate of resistant metal (carborundum). Similar to luminous heat generators, infrared generators are marketed in small units, drawing 50 to 300 watts of power, and large units drawing up to 1500 watts. Reflectors with suitable sockets usually allow the interchangeable use of incandescent bulbs and heating elements of similar wattage (Fig. 5–3).

Electric Light Baths. Electric light baths of the upright type consist of a metal or wooden cabinet fitted with a number of incandescent lamps arranged along the inner sides. The lamps are, as a rule, 60-watt bulbs having a carbon or tungsten filament controlled by a number of switches so that some or all of them may be turned on. The cabinet should be partially open at the top and should have an air vent, preferably at the center of the floor. A thermometer emerging from the top registers the temperature inside.

Energy Emission and Penetration. Heat lamps emit about 95 per cent infrared, 4.8 per cent visible, and 0.1 per cent ultraviolet radiation; the ultraviolet is absorbed by ordinary glass. The wavelength of the infrared extends from 800 to 4,000 millimicrons, with a maximum emission from 800 to 1,600 millimicrons. A similar spectral distribution is obtained with the quartz infrared lamp.

Nonluminous sources emit radiation throughout the entire infrared spectrum to 15,000 millimicrons. The quality of radiation varies according to the surface temperature of the heating element. At the usual in-

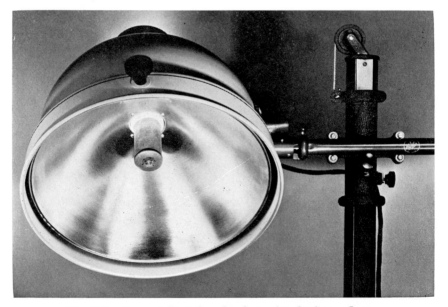

Fig. 5–3. Nonmetallic infrared radiator (Zoalite) in reflector.
(Courtesy of Burdick Corporation.)

tensity, the emission consists principally of the shorter wavelengths, from 2,000 to 3,000 millimicrons.

In recent years, much effort has been spent to evaluate measurements of the *quantity of infrared radiation* emitted from various sources and to clarify the coverage patterns produced by infrared generators and thus allow quantitative prescription of infrared radiation instead of the generally practiced procedure of employing the radiation at a distance of "comfortable tolerance." Because there is no definite beam of radiation, as in roentgen rays, definition of quantity of radiation is replaced by specification of radiation flux, *i.e.*, flow of energy coming from all directions that passes across a unit area of the patient's skin per unit time. This tells how much radiant energy the skin actually receives. A suitable unit for measurement of radiation flux is g cal/cm^2/min. The actual magnitude of the radiation flux at a particular point on the skin will depend not only on the distance of that point from each radiating element of the source (filament, envelope of bulb and reflector) but also on the orientation of the skin to those elements.

The *penetration of infrared rays* has been studied for many years. As already stated in the preceding chapter, any radiation directed to the body may be transmitted unchanged, reflected from its surface, or absorbed and converted back into heat. The penetration of infrared rays depends on their wavelength.

The *difference in penetration* is defined as follows: A radiator operating at relatively low temperature emits long wavelengths that are absorbed primarily in the stratum corneum of the skin; a generator at high temperature, such as the tungsten filament lamp, emits a predominance of near-infrared and visible radiation. The near-infrared penetrates deeply

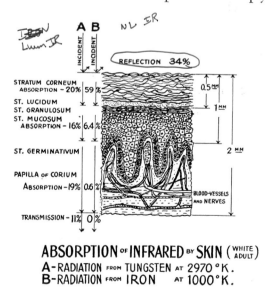

Fig. 5–4. Per cent differential absorption of infrared by skin. (Courtesy of Dr. W. T. Anderson, Jr., and *Archives of Physical Therapy, X-ray and Radium* 18:699, 1937.)

ABSORPTION of INFRARED by SKIN (WHITE ADULT)
A- RADIATION from TUNGSTEN at 2970 °K.
B- RADIATION from IRON at 1000°K.

through skin layers and even into the subcutaneous layers of fat and muscles. The quartz infrared generator has maximum energy in the near-infrared at about 1,500 mμ, giving good penetration and both superficial and relatively deep heating effect, depending on the length of time of the application. Its radiation would penetrate as deeply as that of the tungsten filament lamp. In actual practice, however, the various types of infrared radiators are being used almost interchangeably because much of the effect of infrared radiation is due to reflex effect, for which no deep penetration is necessary.

The depth of penetration is a relative term, whether one means penetration to a depth where the intensity is reduced to 1/10 or 1/10,000 of the incident radiation; and this, in turn depends on the threshold of the biologic effect sought, such as photochemical action or temperature sensation. Small amounts of radiation may penetrate deeper than indicated, but there is insufficient energy at these depths to produce effective biologic action (Fig. 5–4). Authorities differ regarding the transparency of the skin, muscles, tendons, and the like and hence, regarding the depth to which radiation of different wavelengths can penetrate into the body. Transmission measurements seem to indicate that the depth of penetration is not so great as formerly supposed. Furthermore, with increased knowledge of radiation therapy, less emphasis is being placed on this question.

Red glass bulbs in luminous sources of radiation have caused some confusion as to the wavelengths transmitted and their penetration. The glass of the bulb lamp absorbs about 3 per cent of the energy. This amount is not entirely lost, for this energy actually aids in warming the glass, which then radiates energy in the far-infrared field. When a red glass bulb lamp is used, the original radiation is in the infrared part of the spectrum from 700 to 2,000 mμ, with the heated glass itself radiating in the very long-wavelength infrared. The red glass bulb actually radiates less of the infrared rays than the clear glass, but this is of more theoretical than practical interest. The advantage of the colored glass is chiefly that there is less light glare.

PHYSIOLOGICAL EFFECTS OF INFRARED AND LUMINOUS RADIATION

Physiological Effects of Infrared Radiation. Heating the superficial tissues of the body by infrared radiation exerts local as well as general effects; these effects vary according to the extent of the area exposed and the intensity of radiation. There is often an interplay between local and general action. From the clinical standpoint, two main local effects of heat radiation are the stimulation of local circulation and the stimulation of the nerve endings of the skin.

Effect on Circulation. Within a few minutes after exposure to radiant heating, the skin turns red and feels hot; there is no latent period as there is with ultraviolet radiation. The resulting erythema appears in the form of red spots or a network of red lines; it persists, depending on the length of exposure, from 10 minutes up to 1 hour. This erythema is due to the stimulation of the vasomotor mechanism and manifests itself by active vasodilatation of the capillaries and subsequent increase of arterial and venous circulation. There exists an inherent tone in the capillaries that causes vasoconstriction, and the application of heat produces a release of active vasodilator substance. Upon the absorption of the vasodilator substance, more capillaries become active and more blood is supplied to the part.

The erythema caused by dilatation of the capillaries in the corium of the skin occurs after exposure to any form of infrared radiation; in addition, luminous sources containing a large amount of the more penetrating infrared cause a marked stimulation of the sweat glands located in the subcutaneous tissue; as a result, drops of perspiration soon appear in the area under exposure. This effect becomes especially evident when large areas of the skin are exposed to general heat radiation from incandescent sources, as in an electric light cabinet.

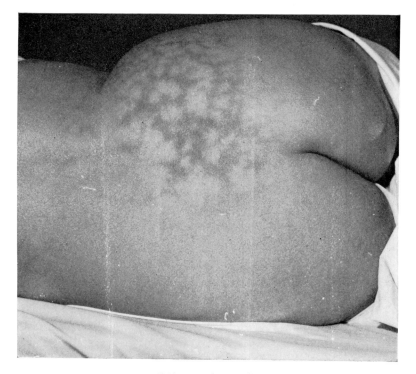

Fig. 5–5. Erythema ab igne.

Table 5–1. Comparison of Infrared and Ultraviolet Rays

	Infrared		Ultraviolet	
Radiation	*Long*	*Short*	*Long*	*Short*
Wavelength	12,000 to 1,600 mμ	1,500 to 700 mμ	400 to 290 mμ	290 to 180 mμ
Penetration	0.1 to 3 mm	10 to 30 mm	0.3 to 0.5 mm	0.1 to 0.3 mm
Erythema { Development	Immediately		After hours (latency)	
Appearance	Darker red, spots or network		Lighter red, sharply bordered	
Duration	Less than one hour		Hours and days	
Pigmentation	Mottled		Homogeneous (tanning)	
Tolerance	Develops occasionally		Increases constantly	

Repeated exposure to infrared radiation may lead to permanent *pigmentation*, which, in contrast to the homogeneous tanning following ultraviolet radiation, is always mottled, like the surface of a marble. The mottled appearance of the skin in regions habitually exposed to heat radiation is called *erythema ab igne* (Fig. 5–5).

Table 5–1 shows a comparison of infrared and ultraviolet radiation, with special reference to erythema production, pigmentation, and tolerance.

Excessive infrared radiation or special sensitivity of the patient results in wheal formation, local edema, and eventually in blistering. Careless exposure may cause deep sloughing, not only in the skin but also in adjacent subcutaneous and fibrous structures.

Effect on Nerve Endings of the Skin. Mild heating results in sedation or relief of pain, while strong heat stimuli cause marked counterirritation. Maximum tolerable surface temperatures are given in Table 5–2. The mechanism of counterirritation may be explained by the desensitization of superficial sensory nerves or by a considerable increase of the stimuli that pass over them: The effect is that of relief of local painful stimuli as well as of those originating from deeper parts and possessing the same nerve center as the area of the skin under the influence of heat. Aside from these two groups of effects explainable by the local thermal effects on tissues, there is no evidence of any specific action of infrared rays; neither is there any evidence of antagonism between these rays and visible or ultraviolet rays in regard to biological effect. There is no scientific basis for giving treatment with a dark infrared source for a few minutes, as if it were comparable to a powerful source of ultraviolet rays.

General Effects. Every local application of heat brings about a certain amount of general heating. The local excess heat is taken up by the bloodstream and carried into the general circulation. The temperature-control mechanism of the body will immediately throw off the additional heat by mild perspiration. Intense general heat application from large heating units ("body bakers" or high-wattage lamps or heat cabinets)

Table 5-2. **Maximum Tolerable Surface Temperatures under Radiant Heating**

Radiation	Surface Temperature	Undersurface Temperature
Short infrared and visible	110.8° F	117.8° F
Long infrared	113.9° F	107.0° F

stimulates the heat-regulating mechanism to full activity in its endeavors to make the output of heat equal that of the increased input.

The generally recognized effects of mild general body heating are: (1) Increased heat elimination and profuse perspiration; (2) increased circulation, a rise of the pulse rate in the ratio of about 10 beats for each degree Fahrenheit, just as occurs in fever; (3) a lowering of blood pressure (in contrast to the effects of cold); (4) increased respiration; (5) increased elimination through the kidneys. There is a loss of water, salt, and urea and other nitrogenous substances, with a relative excess of alkali remaining in the blood and in the tissues, while there is also a temporary loss of body weight. General nervous sensibility is usually markedly lessened.

Physiological Effects of Visible Radiation. Visible radiation is present in all radiation from incandescent sources and from carbon arc and mercury vapor lamps, but its total quantity is relatively small (5 to 15 per cent); the thermal effects of radiation from these sources are attributable principally to the near (short) infrared rays. The generally accepted conception of the physics of visible radiation in relation to the tissues is as follows: 11 per cent of the visible radiation from a tungsten filament lamp is absorbed by the glass bulb, and 33 per cent is reflected by the skin; all of the remainder is absorbed by the superficial layers of the skin but does not penetrate as deeply as the short infrared.

Tyndall demonstrated by classical experiments that it is possible to convert light into heat and *vice versa*. He passed a beam of electric light through water to absorb the heat rays, and then, by passing the resultant rays through a lens of ice, he set fire to black paper, and ignited gun cotton on the other side of the ice, showing that this result was brought about by the light rays exclusively.

There is some justification for the statement that life on this planet is made possible only by visible light. All animal life is ultimately maintained only by vegetation, and formation of plants is based on photosynthesis of carbohydrates from carbon dioxide by chlorophyll under the influence of green light. Knowledge of physiological effects of visible light rays is rather fragmentary. Visible light penetrates into the skin and subcutaneous tissues, and the absorbed energy is transformed into heat and acts in the same way as infrared radiation.

The totality of the visible spectrum may be broken up by prisms or suitable filters into different wavelengths representing different colors. It has been claimed that after separating the visible white into its component parts (red, yellow, blue, etc.) the colored bands can be utilized for specific therapeutic purposes, such as blue for sedation and red for stimulation. There is no evidence to substantiate these claims, chiefly because the filter arrangements for the production of such pure blue, red, or other light, if effective physically, usually weaken the radiation by keeping off the bulk of the electromagnetic energy. Different colors of light undoubtedly exert a certain amount of psychological effect irrespective of the amount of effective radiation.

CLINICAL USE OF LOCAL HEAT RADIATION

Luminous and nonluminous sources of heat radiation produce marked hyperemia, tissue relaxation, and relief of pain in an irradiated area. These effects will assist in the resorption of products of trauma and inflammatory reaction and aid the natural forces of defense and restoration.

The advantages of heat radiation over methods of conductive heating (hot-water bottles, hot packs, etc.) are (1) that its action extends to a greater depth; (2) that there is no pressure over the parts; and (3) that the parts may be kept under constant observation without difficulty. Thus, signs of undue heating can be discovered immediately.

Infrared radiation, on account of its comparative simplicity and safety of application, is preferable to diathermy in many conditions when efficient heating of structures not too deeply situated is desirable. Figure 5–4, showing the penetration of human tissues by the various wavelengths of therapeutic radiation, demonstrates that near infrared penetrates the entire thickness of the skin, part of the subcutaneous tissue, the superficial strata of muscles, and accessible tendons and bones.

The *indications* for the clinical use of infrared heating overlap those for use of heat from conductive and conversive sources. The choice of method depends partly on clinical experience and partly on which method is more easily available. No hard and fast rule exists that would make the selection of a particular form of heating imperative in a given condition.

The principal indication for radiant heating is the relief of pain in the following conditions:

1. Subacute and chronic traumatic and inflammatory conditions in locations accessible to external heating: contusions and muscle strains, traumatic synovitis and tenosynovitis, sprains, dislocations, and fractures.

2. Various forms of arthritis and rheumatoid conditions, neuritis, and neuralgia; in acute forms, mild infrared radiation may be the only means of relieving pain without medication. In these conditions, the advantage over hot packs and hot-water bottles is especially evident because of the avoidance of pressure.

3. Acute, subacute, and chronic catarrhal conditions of the mucous membranes in accessible location: conjunctivitis, coryza, sinusitis.

4. Circulatory disturbances of the extremities (thromboangiitis obliterans, thrombophlebitis, endarteritis obliterans, Raynaud's disease, and erythromelalgia)· Great caution is always needed, and thermostatically controlled heating (kept around 97° F) is safer.

5. Infections of the skin, folliculitis, furunculosis, and even extended abscess formation in the skin. Efficient infrared application may in minor cases reduce the necessity for surgical intervention in the form of incision and drainage. (Hot soaks in early infection hasten localization and are particularly applicable to open wounds, for they loosen crusts and tissue debris and favor removal of dead tissue, thus encouraging drainage). Infrared radiation is convenient to maintain the required temperature in hot antiseptic dressings in infections and cellulitis. It offers the advantage that the heat is constant and is applied without pressure; there is no carrying of infection as may be the case with water; furthermore, the patient need not be disturbed and does not need so much attention. Such radiation, particularly from a luminous source, is often helpful in drying up the exudate of decubitus ulcers when applied for 10 to 15 minutes. Dangers of burns in paraplegic patients must be recognized and guarded against.

6. Radiant heating may be applied as a preliminary to other physical measures. Massage, voluntary and passive exercise, and passive muscular exercise by low-frequency currents should be preceded by some form of heating; the relaxation and preliminary warming makes the tissues supple for manipulation or exercise. Radiant heat is most efficient for this purpose. Preceding the application of the galvanic current with a few minutes' exposure to radiant heat will improve skin conductivity by inducing hyperemia and slight perspiration, thus reducing electrical resistance of the skin.

Choice between Luminous and Nonluminous Radiators. While the quality and penetrating power of the radiation from these two types of generators differ considerably, there are as yet no reliable clinical data to indicate any preference in routine application of radiant heat therapy· It has been stated that the difference between the output of high-temperature (luminous) and low-temperature (nonluminous) radiators is the predominance of the short, more penetrating infrared rays in the first group. More of the long infrared (nonpenetrating) radiation from nonluminous radiators is absorbed by the top layers of the skin, and for this reason such generators feel hotter from the same distance than luminous heat generators of the same wattage and with the same type of reflector.

Individual preferences of patients sometimes favor one source over the other. Patients at times are bothered by a bright light, whereas the dull glow of a lower-temperature generator feels more comfortable. This is especially the case when the face is treated, as in Bell's palsy, and also

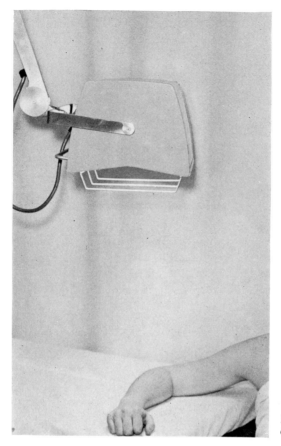

Fig. 5–6.   Luminous heat to elbow (quartz infrared lamp).

in feverish, restless children. There are also some indications that in acute painful conditions radiation from a nonluminous source often feels more soothing. Luminous heating has also proven more effective in conditions where rapid perspiration is desirable. One distinct advantage of a luminous source of radiation is that maximum temperature of the bulb is reached instantaneously, whereas nonluminous heaters need 10 to 15 minutes to obtain operating temperature of the generators.

Technique of Local Radiant Heat Application.   The patient should be placed in a comfortable, relaxed position, and the radiation from the generator directed over the part to be treated at a distance at which it feels comfortable (Fig. 5–6). The distance will average from 2 to 3 feet, according to the sensitivity of the parts, the intensity of the radiation, and the type of reflector. Studies have shown that most of the luminous heat lamps could be applied at distances of 14 to 18 inches. It was also noted that the metal-resistance type of lamp produced some pain at these distances, even though the skin temperature was not raised to the level obtained with the tungsten filament lamps.

Exposure is continued for from 10 to 15 minutes when the object is merely to warm up the parts preliminary to some form of treatment and for 20 to 30 minutes, if heat radiation is the main part of the treatment. The routine employment of a time clock for exact measurement of the time of treatment serves as a protection for patient and physician. Too long exposure, if not too intense, usually does not produce harmful effects in local treatments; in some acute painful conditions, such as brachial neuritis, it may be helpful to apply infrared radiation for as long as one to two hours at a time.

While in most instances infrared radiation should be applied to the bare skin, sheets, towels or other materials are occasionally placed over the part being treated. When applying infrared radiation to the face as in Bell's palsy or sinusitis, the eyes should be protected by moist cotton pledgets. This is to protect the retina from the burning effect of infrared radiation. Patients, too, when administering treatment in their homes often keep on their clothes as a matter of convenience. Various textile materials such as blankets, towels, and cotton and linen sheets transmit 20 to 30 per cent of the long infrared rays and 30 to 40 per cent of the short infrared rays. However, it must not be assumed that the patient will receive only, say, 25 per cent of the energy incident on the upper surface of the blanket. In addition, the blanket will gradually warm up to a temperature determined by the particular circumstances and will transmit energy, not only by secondary radiation, but also by conduction, both by direct contact and across air pockets trapped between the blanket and skin.

Dangers and Precautions.   Exposure to infrared or visible radiation results normally in an erythemal response consisting of individual dark red spots or a confluent network of these spots and occurs according to the distance from the lamp, the wattage of the bulb, the type of reflector, and the sensitivity of the patient. Excess radiation, hypersensitivity, or other causes may produce, after the initial erythema, wheal formation, local edema, and eventually blistering. Sometimes these blisters develop only overnight. Excess radiation in normal patients always gives rise to a varying degree of burning sensation. Special precautions are imperative in patients whose skin sensation is impaired, in those with scars on the skin after burns or other injuries that have destroyed part of the normal skin or its nerve endings, and in patients with peripheral nerve injuries and syringomyelia (Fig. 5–7).

Severely debilitated patients and the elderly tolerate heat poorly. Patients receiving radiation with x rays for malignant disease must not be treated with thermal radiation.

If at any time during treatment the patient complains of unpleasant burning over the entire area or over one spot, the heat lamp should be moved a few inches farther away; this process may have to be repeated until the patient feels entirely comfortable. Patients who receive treat-

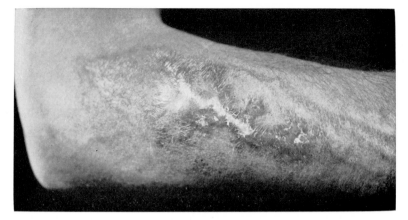

Fig. 5–7.   Scar of burn from infrared lamp in patient with syringomyelia.

ment for the first time often think that a severe burning sensation is part of the treatment; such patients may become blistered, so special watch-fulness is always indicated when treatment is applied for the first time.

Anesthetic areas in patients with peripheral nerve injuries and over scars are especially prone to blister, so in these cases heat generators should be kept at least one and a half times farther away; even then, one should always watch for signs of possible blistering.

Some patients will feel an increase of pain after a 15- to 20-minute local heat application. This is true in acute bursitis and during the first 48 hours after trauma. Increased swelling is thought to be responsible.

CLINICAL USE OF GENERAL BODY HEATING

Indications.   The effects of mild systemic heating on metabolism, on the circulation, and as a sedative led to its clinical employment as a valuable adjunct to general therapeutic measures. General body heating was used especially in chronic stages of venereal diseases before the advent of antibiotics. Today it is used primarily in chronic arthritis and rheumatoid conditions and psychoneuroses—in combination with hydri-atic measures.

Technique.   The technique of general heating by large-wattage heat lamps or infrared radiators is the same as in local heating, save for the larger surface exposed. Applications from 15 minutes to ½ hour at a dis-tance of comfortable toleration are administered.

In electric light cabinets, the lights should be turned on to raise the inside temperature before the patient enters the cabinet. The patient arrives covered by a large sheet or thin bathgown; the covering is then discarded and the patient is seated on a low stool. The top of the cabinet is closed so that the head remains outside. The forehead is covered by

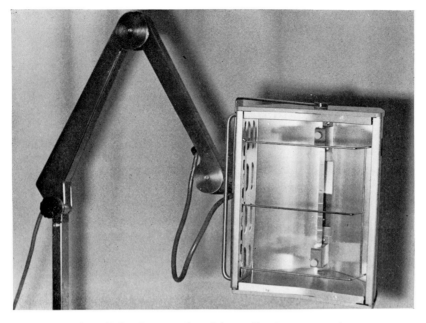

Fig. 5–8. Quartz infrared lamp (luminous source).

a cold-water compress; this prevents headache and too much flushing of the face. If the purpose of the bath is to promote elimination, the patient may drink freely during the treatment in order to encourage perspiration. The patient should never be left alone, and if at any time he feels faint or the pulse rate rises above 100 or becomes irregular, the treatment must be stopped. There are cabinets in which patients can recline, such as fever cabinets, and they are quite convenient for mild general heating. Sauna baths are popular for producing mild elevations of body temperature.

In the light bath thus administered, as a rule, an immediate hyperemia of the skin occurs; there is also a gradual onset of perspiration. The pulse, temperature, and respiration rise in a degree varying with the length of the bath and the individual reaction. As a result, all metabolic and vital activities are quickened.

The duration of the light bath should depend on the desired effect. If general tonic action is desired, the exposure should be brief, 5 to 8 minutes, just to the point of beginning good perspiration.

After the bath the patient should receive a tepid shower or a contrast hot-and-cold (Scotch) douche, according to the stimulation desired; or at least a good rubdown should be given with warm towels or with alcohol. A dry garment is then put on and the patient allowed to rest for 20 to 40 minutes. No patient may leave after a light bath until he has thoroughly cooled off. Baths for tonic purposes may be administered every day or every other day.

In *bedridden patients* general light baths may be administered by suitable electric light bakers.

ADDITIONAL READING

Smithsonian Treasury of Science. Simon & Schuster, New York, 1960, p. 222.

Stone, E. K.: Luminous and infrared heating, pp. 252–265. In S. Licht (ed.), *Therapeutic Heat and Cold*. 2nd ed. Waverly Press, Baltimore, 1965.

Stillwell, G. K.: Therapeutic heat, pp. 233–243. In F. H. Krusen, F. J. Kottke, and P. M. Ellwood (eds.), *Handbook of Physical Medicine and Rehabilitation*. W. B. Saunders Co., Philadelphia, 1965.

PART III

Ultraviolet Radiation

Chapter 6

PHYSICS AND EFFECTS

Generation. Very hot bodies and ionized gases emit ultraviolet rays. In order to obtain an appreciable amount of ultraviolet radiation, it is necessary to heat the radiating substance to a temperature of 3000° C (5400° F) or higher (Coblentz). The chief natural source of ultraviolet radiation is the sun. The sources of artificial ultraviolet radiation are chiefly electric arcs between electrodes of metals and of carbon and of mercury in quartz. Radiations from artificial sources represent only approximations to sunlight, and no two are alike in respect to the spectral distribution of the energy they emit.

Classification. The range of radiant energy designated as ultraviolet extends from 390 to 180 millimicrons and is divided into (1) "near ultraviolet" radiation, which is contiguous to the luminous rays and consists of comparatively long rays, extending downward to 290 millimicrons; and (2) "far ultraviolet" radiation, consisting of comparatively short rays, extending from 290 to 180 millimicrons wavelength (Fig. 6–1). The sun's spectrum contains none of these short rays, since the earth's atmosphere filters them out before they reach sea level.

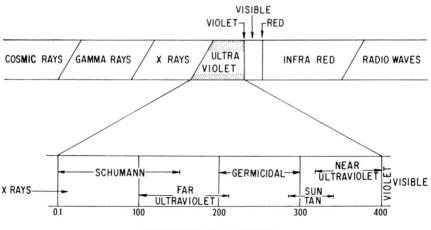

Fig. 6–1. Electromagnetic spectrum (enlargement of ultraviolet region). (Courtesy of GTE Sylvania Incorporated.)

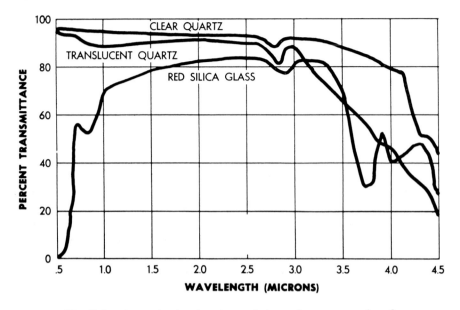

Fig. 6–2. Approximate glass transmission values vs. wavelength. (Courtesy of GTE Sylvania Incorporated.)

Physical Properties. Ultraviolet rays penetrate to a very limited extent through bodies. Quartz permits their passage down to 180 mμ, hence the employment of quartz for the construction of burners and filters. Ordinary window glass permits only the passage of rays longer than 320 millimicrons (see Fig. 6–2).

The human skin arrests all ultraviolet radiation, and beyond the depth of 2 mm only the rays longer than 450 mμ can penetrate. Paper and even the thinnest underwear arrest most of the radiation.

Penetration. According to the law of Grotthuss, formulated in 1819, only the rays that are absorbed are physiologically active. Painstaking studies in recent years have established the transmission of various forms of radiant energy through the skin.

The human skin consists of two principal layers, the outer skin or epidermis and the dermis or corium (Figs. 6–3 and 6–4). In the outer skin there is the horny layer or corneum with flat epithelial cells, the transitional layer of granulosum with flat granular cells, and the stratum spinosum, with the basal layer and pigment cells. In the dermis, there is a papillary layer or rete vasculosum containing nerve terminals and vessels and a reticular layer. Below the two layers of the skin is the subcutaneous tissue mainly consisting of fat. Radiant energy penetrates through these layers differently according to its wavelength and exerts physiological effects in the layer where it is absorbed.

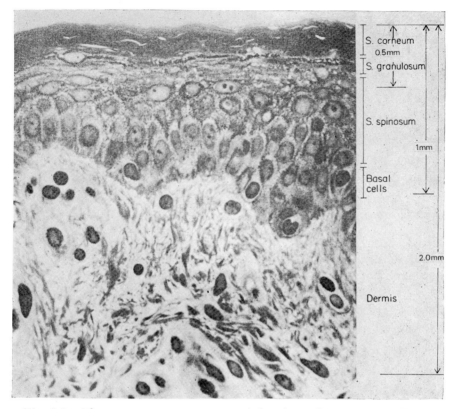

S. corneum
0.5mm
S. granulosum

S. spinosum

1mm

Basal
cells

2.0mm

Dermis

Fig. 6–3. Electron microscopic structure of skin (×800). Compare with Figure 6–4, p. 44. (From Odland and Short, 1971, reprinted with permission of McGraw-Hill Book Company.)

A summary of the penetration, absorption and relative energy transmission of radiant energy in the human skin is as follows:

Far infrared: Practically no penetration.

Near infrared: Strongly increasing absorption in upper layers, decreasing in lower layers.

Visible: Minimum absorption in stratum corneum. Most radiation absorbed in dermis.

Pronounced radiation of both visible and infrared radiation reaches subcutaneous layers.

Near ultraviolet: Relatively large absorption in stratum spinosum.

Far ultraviolet: Greatest absorption in stratum corneum. Some radiation reaches corium (papillare).

No radiation of near ultraviolet or far ultraviolet reaches subcutaneous layers.

Extreme ultraviolet: All absorbed by corneum. No radiation reaching basal cell layer.

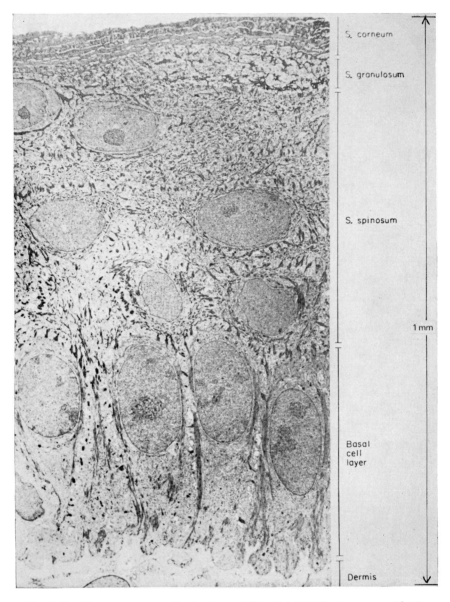

S. corneum

S. granulosum

S. spinosum

1 mm

Basal
cell
layer

Dermis

Fig. 6–4. Electron microscopic structure of skin (× 2,900). Compare with Figure 6–3, p. 43. (From Odland and Short, 1971, reprinted with permission of McGraw-Hill Book Company.)

Table 6–1. Comparative Physical Effects of Radiation

Mainly thermal	Infrared	Little effect on the photographic plate / Strong heating effects
	Red	Fairly marked heating effects
	Yellow	Fairly marked luminous effects
Luminous	Green	Little heating
	Violet	Very little heat effect / Marked luminous effects / Marked effects in photography
Mainly chemical	Ultraviolet	Marked effects in photography

Comparative Physical Effects. Although we can sharply differentiate between infrared, visible, and ultraviolet radiation from a standpoint of physical measurements, on the borderline between these different wavelengths, no such sharp demarcation occurs, from the standpoint of either physical or physiological effects. Table 6–1 shows the gradual merging of the physical effects of infrared (thermal), luminous, and ultraviolet (photochemical) radiation.

Comparative Physiological Effects. Radiant energy when absorbed by the tissue cells brings about a complex variety of physical, chemical, and biological reactions. From the standpoint of physical therapy, we may divide radiant energy into photothermal and photochemical radiations.

Photothermal radiations, comprising infrared and visible radiation, penetrate subcutaneous tissues, heat the blood, accelerate vital reactions, and act instantaneously; they produce a burning sensation or immediate burn when their intensity is too great. By reflex, effects on pain and circulation in deeper structures can be elicited. (See Table 6–2.)

Photochemical radiations, comprising ultraviolet radiation, penetrate only to fractions of millimeters; they are absorbed by protoplasm, and this absorption results in physical and biological changes that manifest themselves only several hours after exposure. Thermal radiations are employed more often for immediate local action, while photochemical radiations are used more frequently for their secondary or subsequent effect on the general organism. (See Table 6–2.)

The therapeutic importance of the ultraviolet part of radiant energy has received considerably less attention in recent years, and the tremendous value of the longer spectral wavelengths has not received the consideration it deserves. Visible and infrared radiation are at least equally essential for all organic life. It has been stated that if the heat rays of the sun were to be screened off the earth, it would be surrounded by an ice crust in short order. Likewise, if the sun were to cease sending us the green portion of the spectrum, on which depends the formation of chlorophyll—all-important for plant life—most life on earth would become extinct. Just

Table 6–2. Different Spectral Regions, Probable Depth of Penetration, and Probable Physiologic Action of Rays from Different Sources[a]

Spectral Region	Penetration of Rays	Physiologic Action	Source
Far ultraviolet 180 to 290 mμ	Superficial 0.01 to 0.1 mm	Photochemical	Metals in carbon arc and spark of metals (mercury arc)
Near ultraviolet 290 to 390 mμ	Superficial 0.1 to 1 mm	Photochemical	Sun; metals in carbon arc; arc of metals
Visible spectrum 390 to 760 mμ	Deep 1 to 10 mm	Thermal; nerve stimulation	Sun, carbon arc
Near infrared 760 to 1,500 mμ	Deep 1 to 10 mm	Thermal; nerve stimulation	Sun; carbon arc; gas-filled tungsten lamp and carbon filament incandescent lamp, rods
Far infrared 1,500 to 15,000 mμ	Superficial 1 to 0.05 mm	Thermal; nerve stimulation	Infrared heaters

[a] From Coblentz and Stair.

as normal organic life demands an unbroken supply of all of the rays of the solar spectrum, so in therapy, infrared and luminous radiation play an essential role in many of the results of the application of radiant energy.

Ultraviolet radiation brings about fluorescence of many substances. The surface of a roentgen-ray screen becomes phosphorescent after exposure to ultraviolet rays. They exert photochemical effects in decomposing silver salts and in discoloring vegetable colors and photoelectric effects causing emission of electrons from negatively charged metals. If a negatively charged electroscope is placed in the path of certain ultraviolet rays, its leaves collapse, showing the loss of its electric charge. The presence of ultraviolet rays in any light can be proved by this simple test. The formation of ozone from the oxygen of the air by photosynthesis is also attributed to the action of ultraviolet rays. Ozone has a characteristic odor easily recognized by the physical therapist.

PHYSIOLOGICAL EFFECTS OF ULTRAVIOLET RADIATION

The variety of effects of ultraviolet radiation on substances outside of the human organism points to the possibility of much more complex effects on the intricate tissues in the living organism. The fundamental principles of the biophysics and physiology of radiation are still unsolved, and the real action of radiation on the living cell is unknown.

Ultraviolet light does not act as a unit biologically, for various parts of the large ultraviolet spectrum cause different biological effects. The very long wavelengths (from about 320 to 310 mμ) penetrate deeper into the skin, but exert little biological action; the very short rays (below 230 mμ) have practically no penetration and also exert very little biological effect; it is in the intervening wavelength zone from about 310 to 250 millimicrons where most of the biological reactions occur. Some of these zones or bands have very distinct effects, and some generators are being developed that produce so-called "monochromatic" radiation.

The effects of ultraviolet radiation from a biological standpoint have been classified as photochemical ones occurring in the skin and biological ones occurring in the blood and in the metabolism. The photochemical effect ends with the production of dermatitis and the activation of substances in the skin and possibly in the blood, while the biological, the effect on metabolism, growth, circulation, and so on, lasts for some time.

From the therapeutic standpoint, the physiological action of ultraviolet may be discussed under the headings of erythema production, pigmentation, bactericidal effects, antirachitic effects, and, finally, effects on the blood and metabolism.

Erythema Production. Radiant energy between wavelengths of 320 and 240 millimicrons produces local erythema of the skin which develops in 2 to 8 hours, depending on the sensitivity of the subject and on the intensity of the radiation. Because this effect appears most rapidly and is among the easiest to detect, it has come to be considered as a sign of an effective light source or as a measure of an effective dose of radiation.

Degrees of Erythema. Erythema of the skin is a true inflammatory reaction and can be described according to its intensity, as of four different degrees. Each of these degrees is associated with the conception of a definite dosage of ultraviolet radiation:

(*a*) Minimal erythema dose (also called first-degree and tonic dose): A reaction so slight that it is scarcely noticed by the patient. The skin reddening is very faint, occurs after a latent period of some 6 to 8 hours, and usually subsides within 24 to 36 hours without leaving any trace whatsoever. Should be administered on the entire body or largest possible area. A reaction just below the minimal erythema is called a suberythemal dose.

(*b*) Second-degree erythema: A mild sunburn reaction. The reddening is plainly visible after 4 to 6 hours and is followed on subsidence by slight desquamation. Subsides in about 2 days and may leave some pigmentation.

(*c*) Third-degree erythema, also designated as a counterirritant dose: An intense reaction similar to sunburn. The reddening is intense after 3 to 4 hours, and there is also a slight edema. It may be followed by peeling of the skin and takes about three days to subside, leaving pigmentation. This sunburn is essentially employed as a local reaction.

(*d*) Fourth-degree erythema, also designated as a destructive dose: An intense reddening, supervening after a short latent period (about 2 hours) and increasing until exudation and blistering results; persists for many days and is followed by peeling. Administered only on small areas, at contact, or short distance.

Histological Changes. The histological changes associated with erythema production are as follows: The capillary vessels of the irradiated area are dilated and filled with red blood cells. With an increase in permeability, a transudate of plasma proteins occurs. There is marked leukocytosis in the irradiated area, and this reaction is not confined to the irradiated surface but extends deep into the tissues. It can be seen as early as 30 minutes after ultraviolet exposure and becomes maximal between 8 and 24 hours. Following intense irradiation, there is serofibrinous and often hemorrhagic exudation, and in a further stage thrombi form in the vessels of the arteries, and degeneration and necrosis of the skin as well as of the deeper parts may follow. The prickle cell layer absorbs the light, and protein is denatured and the cell is damaged. Vasodilator substance diffuses to subdermal levels, where it causes a vasodilatation. A phase of regeneration begins after 96 hours. With the routine mild erythema doses, however, the usual reaction is a dilatation of the superficial vessels with some increase in blood flow; after a duration of the hyperemia for a varying period, there is full restoration to normal.

Hyperplasia. It is well known that the epidermis of human skin that has been exposed to solar radiation becomes thicker. In the first 24 to 48 hours, there is an apparent increase in thickness of epidermis due to intercellular and intracellular edema. Within 72 hours of exposure, hyperplasia is visible microscopically and is indicated by increase in mitosis. By 72 hours, the increase in mitotic rate is maximum. All layers of the epidermis except the basal layer are thickened.

The spinosum layer reaches maximum thickness in a week. The rate of proliferation of cells falls off after 7 to 10 days, and the thickness of the epidermis gradually returns to normal within the next 30 to 60 days if the skin remains unexposed.

Difference in Erythema Effect of Certain Wavelengths. No perceptible erythemal effect is produced by wavelengths below 240 or above 320 millimicrons. The almost immediate reddening of the skin after irradiation by a strong source of mixed radiation such as the sun or a heat lamp or carbon arc lamp is due to radiant heat rays. Such reddening is not restricted to the irradiated parts of the skin, has a mottled appearance, and disappears soon after irradiation has stopped.

Within the range of wavelengths with erythemal action, there are two maximal areas of erythemal effectiveness, as shown in Figure 6–5. One is at about 300 millimicrons, the other at about 250 millimicrons. These two maxima have not the same value in a photobiological sense. Erythema produced by radiation at 300 millimicrons is followed, according to its intensity, by strong pigmentation and painful blistering—a real sunburn—while erythema produced by radiation around 250 millimicrons leaves scarcely any, or at most only an inconsiderable, pigmentation.

Biological Explanation of Erythema. Research work on the biophysical response of the skin to radiation at different wavelengths has offered an explanation of the diverse erythema and pigmentation action of the two maxima of the erythema curve.

The erythema production of the skin is a true inflammatory reaction and is in degree similar to those described by Lewis as a result of mechanical, thermal or electrical stimuli. After irradiation, the walls of skin vessels become permeable and their cells activated, and certain substances in the skin pass from these cells into the blood. Among the substances affected is the H-substance of Lewis, histidine, which undergoes a photochemical change into histamine. Histamine produces a vivid erythema when introduced into the skin even in minimal amounts. Only wavelengths under 270 mμ bring about this histidine-histamine change; hence the vivid erythemal action of these shorter wavelengths without pigmentation. On the other hand, tyrosine and other amino acids are also activated in the skin by irradiation; tyrosine is the substance that produces pigment that is deposited in the horny layers of the epidermis. Wavelengths of 300 millimicrons bring about this change and hence the tanning effect following erythemal doses of the longer ultraviolet wavelengths. The nature and the mode of this inflammatory response have been the subject of a number of hypotheses; these are discussed by Pathak and Epstein.

Erythema Reaction as a Measure of Effectiveness of Ultraviolet Radiation. While the erythema is by no means the most important biological effect of ultraviolet radiation, it serves at present as the only available practical basis for judging clinically the effectiveness of ultraviolet radiation. Physiatrists have adopted this reaction for the measure of efficiency of ultraviolet generators for two reasons: (1) In the case of exposure to

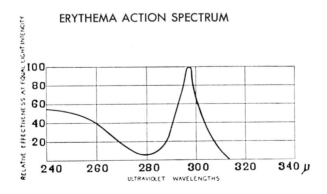

Fig. 6–5. Curve of erythemal effectiveness of radiant energy.

intense sources of ultraviolet radiation, it is a simple and practical means of preventing severe burns. (2) In the case of weak sources of ultraviolet radiation, it is an efficient safeguard against possible fraudulent sale of lamps deficient in ultraviolet radiation.

Pigmentation. Repeated irradiation with erythema doses between 280 and 300 mμ causes pigmentation that consists of a deposit of granules of the pigment melanin in the basal cells of the epidermis. Pigmentation and erythema are associated only in the longer wavelengths, for as already stated, the erythema-producing wavelengths around 250 mμ are not followed by late pigmentation. It is also well known that repeated stimulation by other agents such as repeated friction and other mechanical irritation may also bring about deposition of pigment. Histologically, pigment production is the local response in the epithelial and basal cells of the epidermis. There is definite evidence to indicate that there are two mechanisms producing pigmentation. The first is a general factor, a certain amount of cell proliferation that causes melanin pigment granules, or melanosomes, from the basal layers of the skin to migrate upward. The second appears to be a true photochemical reaction; it occurs chiefly after intense exposure to wavelengths from 320 to 420 mμ, and requires no latent period; it may be interpreted as oxidation of bleached pigment already in the skin from previous tanning. This second mechanism appears to be responsible for the more pronounced tanning of the skin after exposure to sunlight than to artificial sources of light.

It has been shown in subjects exposed to a sunlight lamp (type S-4) at a distance of 2½ feet that the average exposure required to produce a minimal erythema visible one day later was 4 minutes, and a minimal tan visible 2 months later, 7½ minutes. With this lamp, most of the erythema and tan are produced at 296.7 and 302 millimicrons. Except in June, July, and August, tanning by sunlight in the northern hemisphere is possible only between 9:00 A.M. and 3:00 P.M.

The role of pigmentation is not yet fully determined. The melanosomes not only absorb ultraviolet radiations but also scatter them. It is generally accepted that the intensity of pigmentation is an indicator of the action of radiant energy and is proportional to the amount of radiation. But it is also dependent upon individual factors such as race, constitution, and body function. On the other hand, it has been shown that the role of pigmentation in warding off sunburn is only a minor one, and that it is the thickening of the stratum corneum of the skin that mainly affords that protection. This is proven by the fact that the palms of the hands and soles of the feet, which do not tan but where the corneum is the thickest, never suffer a sunburn.

Metabolic Effects. The most spectacular and most intensively studied effects of ultraviolet irradiation occur along photobiochemical lines, especially relating to the metabolism of sterols and the production of vitamin D:

(*a*) *Activation of Vitamin D* (antirachitic effect). Ultraviolet radiation having wavelengths below 320 millimicrons is absorbed by the plant sterol ergosterol and by the 7-D hydrocholesterol contained in the corneum and upper layers of the skin, hair follicles, and sebaceous and sweat glands, and vitamin D is the by-product of this exposure.

The mechanism of this transformation is a complicated biochemical process. Vitamin D is an essential necessity of life; it promotes normal anabolism of calcium and retention of phosphorus. Following ultraviolet irradiation, the calcium content of the blood serum is increased by increased absorption from the intestines of the calcium and phosphate in the food. This effect is vital for the prevention and treatment of rickets and other calcium-deficiency conditions, such as tetany, and also for the development and care of the teeth in the absence of adequate dietary intake of vitamin D. Ultraviolet irradiation of the lactating woman increases, to an extent, the quantity and antirachitic potency of the milk. It also has been found possible to render cow's milk antirachitic by direct irradiation. Milk is the only common food considered for acceptance by the Council on Foods and Nutrition when fortified with vitamin D. The action of ultraviolet and cod-liver oil on calcium and phosphorus retention are interchangeable. One of the newer methods used to impart antirachitic properties to milk is to irradiate cholesterol or ergosterol and add the antirachitic derivative to the milk.

Vitamin D in oral preparations is now so readily available that ultraviolet irradiation from artificial sources is not of clinical significance for its antirachitic effect.

(*b*) *Other Metabolic Changes.* The older literature on ultraviolet radiation is filled with claims of numerous effects on circulating red blood cells and a great variety of metabolic processes. These claims have not been substantiated sufficiently over the years to make them of therapeutic value.

Bactericidal Effects. The lethal effect of ultraviolet radiation on bacteria, viruses, and fungi has been studied extensively in recent years, and it was found that that spectral band at 265.2 mμ produces the maximum bactericidal effect, while that at 253.7 mμ is only 90 per cent effective. This action depends on the disruption of the constituent nucleic acid molecule by absorption of these wavelengths.

Bactericidal effects on the tissues of the human body by ultraviolet are limited by the penetration of ultraviolet to the uppermost layer of the skin—a depth of 2 mm. Most of the standard lamps emit only a limited amount in the bactericidal range and because of the preponderance of the other intense erythema-producing rays, the effective use of the germicidal band is negligible.

In recent years, ultraviolet lamps have been constructed that emit principally bactericidal radiation, and extensive laboratory and clinical studies have been made of the various aspects of such radiation. As a result, ultraviolet air disinfection has been introduced on an industrial scale.

ADDITIONAL READING

Coblentz, W. W., and Stair, R.: J. Nat. Bur. Standards *12*:13, 1934.

Lewis, T.: *The Blood Vessels of the Human Skin and Their Responses.* Shaw and Sons, London, 1927.

Licht, S. H. (ed.): *Therapeutic Electricity and Ultraviolet Radiation.* 2d ed. Licht, New Haven, Conn., 1967.

Luckiesh, M., and Taylor, A. H.: Production of erythema and tan by ultraviolet energy. J.A.M.A. *112*:2511, 1939.

Odland, G. F., and Short, J. M.: Structure of the skin, p. 41. In T. B. Fitzpatrick *et al.* (ed.), *Dermatology in General Medicine.* McGraw-Hill Book Co., New York, 1971.

Pathak, M. A., and Epstein, J. H.: Normal and abnormal reactions of man to light, p. 977. In T. B. Fitzpatrick *et al.* (ed.), *Dermatology in General Medicine.* McGraw-Hill Book Co., New York, 1971.

Urbach, F.: *The Biologic Effects of Ultraviolet Radiation.* Pergamon Press, Oxford, 1969, p. 107.

Chapter 7

ARTIFICIAL ULTRAVIOLET THERAPY

General Considerations. In artificial sources of radiation, there may be considerable difference in the proportion and intensity of the various wavelengths, as indicated in Table 7–1. Furthermore, while we speak of ultraviolet rays, the fact holds that in most instances we are using infrared and visible radiation together with the ultraviolet.

Historical. Artificial light therapy had its inception in Niels Finsen's classical experiments, done in 1893 at Copenhagen, showing that the ultraviolet or chemical rays of sunlight have stimulating and bactericidal effects on lower organisms. Employing carbon arc light, which just then came into use for lighting, he filtered out the heat rays with water and achieved excellent results in the treatment of tuberculosis of the skin (lupus) by concentrated light. The mercury vapor or quartz lamp was developed from the Cooper-Hewitt lamp of 1891, in which mercury vapor was excited by an electrical current for use in lighting. In 1903, Heræus devised tubes from fused quartz that were transparent to ultraviolet rays. Bach and Nagelschmidt developed the quartz mercury vapor lamp for general radiation, and Kromeyer the "water-cooled" mercury vapor lamp for contact treatments. In recent years, many newer, more efficient forms of ultraviolet generators have been developed.

Inasmuch as carbon arc lamps are rarely used therapeutically, the details of their construction, operation, and radiation characteristics will be

Table 7–1. Principal Forms of Phototherapeutic Radiation

Source	Predominant rays	Approximate Wavelengths
Heating elements	Infrared	12,000 to 600 mμ
Incandescent lamps	Infrared and visible	5,000 to 400 mμ
Carbon arcs	Infrared Visible Long ultraviolet	12,000 to 240 mμ
High-amperage mercury arc (hot quartz)	Visible Long and short ultraviolet	3,000 to 200 mμ
High-voltage mercury arc (cold quartz)	Short ultraviolet	Almost all at 250 mμ

omitted. Their usefulness was predicated upon the fact that these lamps gave off a continuous spectrum plus a band spectrum that emphasized areas in the ultraviolet range. Since vitamin D is readily available orally, the antirachitic effects of the carbon arc lamp are no longer of practical importance.

MERCURY VAPOR LAMPS

Mercury, a liquid metal at room temperature, when vaporized in a quartz container by intense heat, emits a spectrum rich in ultraviolet, characterized by a series of intense spectral lines or bands. All electric discharges in mercury vapor produce the mercury spectrum, provided the lamp has an envelope of fused quartz. Quartz or silicon dioxide glass is extremely heat resistant and at the same time freely transmits ultraviolet radiations. Ultraviolet lamps, which have an outer jacket of glass or employ a glass envelope instead of quartz, produce a spectrum of mercury restricted by the transmission characteristics of the glass. The wavelength and flux intensity of these spectral bands vary according to the construction of the generator.

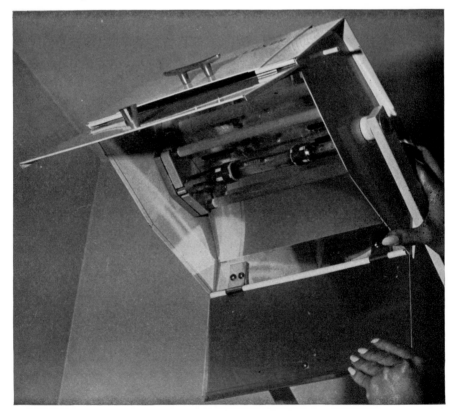

Fig. 7–1. Quartz burner.

The mercury vapor pressure in lamps may fall within three groups: (1) high pressure, of the order of 1 to 10 atmospheres, in hot quartz lamps; (2) medium pressure of the order of 0.1 atmosphere, in moderately warm lamps; and (3) low pressure, of the order of 0.001 atmosphere, in cold quartz lamps.

High-Pressure Mercury Lamps. The principal part of the high-pressure quartz vapor lamps is the "burner," a fused quartz tube, exhausted of air and containing mercury (Fig. 7–1). Suitable attachments conduct an electric current to the burner, which is housed in an adjustable chromium or aluminum reflector. Present types of hot quartz burners usually consist of "activated" tubes filled with argon gas and just a small amount of mercury. They light up without tilting (required for starting the older lamps) as soon as the current is turned on and produce full output within a few minutes.

The emission of the high-pressure mercury lamp contains very little short infrared radiation, a fairly large amount of the violet end of the visible spectrum, and a large amount of ultraviolet; about 6 per cent of the total radiation is of wavelengths shorter than 290 millimicrons, entirely absent in sunlight. *There is considerable difference between this type of radiation and that of the sun.* The spectrogram of the mercury arc consists of a series of spectral lines superimposed on a faint continuous spectrum (Fig. 7–2). The quartz tube and the hood emit a low-temperature, long-wave radiation.

Quartz burners slowly deteriorate with use because the quartz tube decreases in transparency and does not transmit as much of the light as before. The decrease of intensity affects all portions of the spectrum in nearly

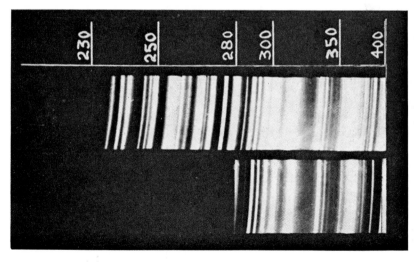

Fig. 7–2. Spectrum of quartz mercury arc through Corex-D glass. Upper photograph shows full spectrum; lower shows only radiation of wavelengths longer than 280 mμ, all short waves having been filtered out.

equal measure. The greatest decrease occurs during the first hundred hours of operation, and it is estimated that after that period the ultraviolet intensity is about 80 per cent of the original one. After 1,000 hours the total intensity of radiation is from two-thirds to one-half of the intensity when new, provided the lamps operate on the same voltage and amperage. Erythema tests should be applied periodically to check efficiency of the burner. The ultraviolet energy output can also be physically measured from time to time.

The burners and lamps illustrated serve chiefly for general irradiation, and since they are kept at a considerable distance from the body, the air circulating under the hood is sufficient to keep the burners from overheating; hence their designation as "air-cooled" lamps (Fig. 7–3). Special mercury vapor lamps designed for local treatment have been earlier known

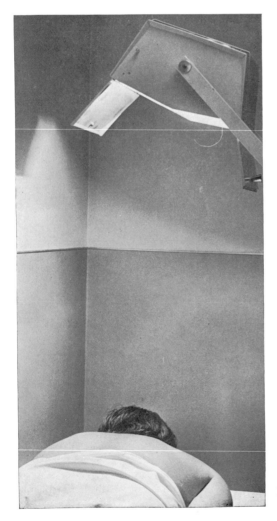

Fig. 7–3. Artificial ultraviolet irradiation.

as "water-cooled" or Kromeyer lamps. In these, the burner was surrounded by a water jacket with inflow and outflow tubes for cold water and had a quartz window at one side for the transmission of radiation from which the heat rays had been absorbed.

The simplicity of handling and upkeep has made the hot quartz lamps the most widely used source of artificial light. They require comparatively little current; any other surce of ultraviolet energy can produce the same intensity of radiation only by the expenditure of much more electrical energy. With suitable "filters," various parts of their spectral emissions can be utilized.

Low-Pressure Quartz Lamps. In these lamps, a narrow quartz tube containing mercury and neon gas is excited by an electrical current of high voltage. A transformer steps up the alternating current supply to about 2500 volts; the amperage and vapor pressure in the glow tube is very low; there is little current consumption, and consequently the tube remains cold and can be readily placed near the body or inserted in orifices (Fig. 7–4). The full energy emission of these lamps is present within a minute of turn-on, and it remains extremely constant.

The spectral emission of low-pressure quartz lamps is largely (about 95 per cent) in the 253 mμ line in the short ultraviolet field. This ultraviolet band has enough penetrating power through the epidermis to cause biological and therapeutic effects; it also is antirachitic in rats, as are all radiations around 250 millimicrons. It produces erythema without much pigmentation or blistering.

The radiations emitted by low-pressure mercury lamps are not encountered in sunlight because they are filtered out by the earth's atmosphere. Thus they are not very useful in studies of sunburn and photosensitivity reactions. The prevalence of bactericidal radiations from these quartz

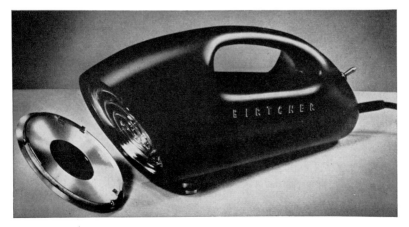

Fig. 7–4. Low-pressure quartz lamp for local application. Equipped with a Wood's filter, it enables fluorescent (black light) examination. (Courtesy of Birtcher Corporation.)

3

generators points to their usefulness in surgical rooms and tissue-culture laboratories. They are used almost exclusively in the present-day method of air disinfection and are marketed under a variety of names, e.g., germicidal lamps.

Fluorescent Sunlamp. These lamps (Fig. 7–5) may be used without a reflector. The 20-watt lamp will produce a minimal erythema at a distance of 2 feet in 20 minutes with the bare lamp and in 7 minutes with a reflector. At the same distance, a 40-watt lamp will produce a minimal erythema in half the time with the bare lamp and with the reflector.

RS (Reflector) Type Sunlamps. These consist of a mercury arc tube enclosed in a special glass bulb (Corex D or a special Corning type), opaque to short-wavelength ultraviolet (below 280 mμ). Some of these lamps also contain ballast coils made of tungsten filament which, when heated, limit the current passing through the mercury arc tube and which then radiates infrared and visible light (Fig. 7–6). The lamps all emit ultraviolet radiation in accordance with the requirements for sunlamps, normally a minimum perceptible erythema in 5 minutes at 24 inches.

The chief advantage of these newer sunlamps is that they can be screwed into any 110- to 125-volt alternating current socket and will burn in any position. They consume from 100 to 275 watts, according to their construction; some of the bulbs are partly coated with aluminum so as to form a reflector.

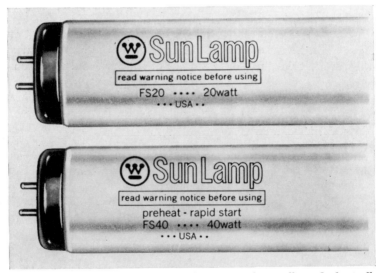

Fig. 7–5. Westinghouse fluorescent sunlamps are electrically and physically identical with regular fluorescent lamps of corresponding wattage. Instead of producing visible light however, they radiate ultraviolet energy. This is accomplished through the use of a special glass tubular bulb whose inside is coated with a special Westinghouse developed phosphor. An electrical discharge within the tube generates 253.7-mμ ultraviolet energy, which excites the white phosphors, causing them to fluoresce and radiate a considerable amount of invisible ultraviolet energy in the 280- to 350-mμ band. (Courtesy of Westinghouse Electric Co.)

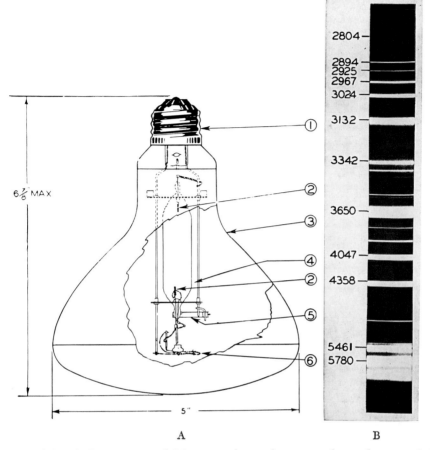

Fig. 7–6. A, Section view of RS-type sunlamp, showing six basic elements: (1) medium screw base, (2) electrodes, in bulb, (3) special ultraviolet-transmitting reflector bulb, (4) quartz arc tube, (5) bimetallic starting switch, and (6) tungsten filament ballast. (Courtesy of Westinghouse Electric Co.) B, Spectral emission (in angstrom units) of above RS-type sunlamp in the ultraviolet region; in addition, there is some infrared emission generated by the tungsten filament ballast.

CHOICE OF ULTRAVIOLET GENERATORS AND STANDARDS OF EMISSION

Our present ultraviolet generators generally furnish combinations of the three principal groups of radiations: (1) infrared, luminous, and full range of ultraviolet radiation, as represented by the modern carbon arc lamp; (2) luminous and partial range of ultraviolet radiation, as represented by the high-pressure quartz lamp; (3) an almost monochromatic radiation of short ultraviolet, as represented by the low-pressure quartz lamp and the air-disinfecting units (Table 7–2 shows the principal sources of phototherapeutic radiation and the spectral range of their emissions);

Table 7–2. Choice of Ultraviolet Generators

Type	Spectral Range	Predominant Radiation
High-pressure quartz	580–185 mμ	Long- and short-wave ultraviolet
Low-pressure quartz	253 mμ	Short-wave ultraviolet

(4) monochromatic generators, which have recently become available for laboratory use.

Standards of Emission. The effectiveness of ultraviolet generators was judged by the Council on Physical Medicine on the basis of the erythemal reaction, and this is still the accepted clinical practice. The specifications of minimum intensity are based on a comfortable and convenient operating distance (24 inches or 61 cm) from the front edge of the reflector, at which distance the exposure can be made without burning the skin by contact with the burner or by the infrared rays. The ultraviolet intensity of the lamp shall be such that the time of exposure to produce a minimum perceptible erythema (one that disappears in less than 24 hours) will not be longer than 15 minutes for a therapeutic lamp and 60 minutes for so-called sunlamps. Modern high-pressure mercury arc lamps for hospital use may produce a minimum perceptible erythema with a 15-second exposure at 30 inches.

As the emission line of the mercury arc lamp of 296 millimicrons has the highest efficiency in generating an erythema, this line appears suited as a natural standard for evaluating sources of heterogeneous ultraviolet radiation. Twenty microwatts per square centimeter of homogeneous radiation of wavelength 296.7 millimicrons has been adopted as the erythemal unit (EU) of dosage; that is, 1 EU = 20 microwatts per square centimeter of radiation of wavelength 296.7 millimicrons. For home use, lamps that emit practically no ultraviolet radiation shorter than 280 millimicrons are recommended.

Lamps for disinfecting purposes require 100 microwatts per square centimeter of homogeneous radiation of wavelength 253.7 mμ as the unit of germicidal intensity. The difference in effectiveness from the 265.2 band is negligible. Since the ultraviolet emission from the low-vapor-pressure mercury discharge tube is practically homogeneous radiation of wavelength 253.7, such a lamp can be readily calibrated in absolute value and used as a standard.

TECHNIQUE OF ULTRAVIOLET IRRADIATION

Administration. In general irradiation, the entire unclothed body is exposed; hence, the treatment room should be warm and also well aired. It is advisable to provide an individual dressing gown or sheet for each patient to cover him until the actual exposure. The eyes of the patient as well as those of the operator should be protected by goggles. Ordinary leatherette goggles can be bought cheaply by the dozen, and individual goggles can be provided for each patient. In patients with a sensitive skin, it may be well to cover the face with a thin towel at first; the genitalia should generally be covered by a loin cloth or a folded towel. A shield cut from heavy paper may protect the nipples. If the face is exposed, it should not rest on a high support, since this would result in a more intense exposure because of the shorter distance from the lamp.

Patients are usually treated in the recumbent position. The table or couch on which the patient rests should be a low one, allowing a ready variation of the distance from the lamp. Modern mercury vapor lamps now allow radiation at various angles instead of only from the horizontal or vertical position. The center part of the body should be placed in the direct line of radiation, but no old-style hot quartz lamp should ever be placed directly over the patient's body.

With the high-pressure mercury vapor lamp, one must wait for 2 minutes or more, according to the type of lamp, until the full output of radiation is developed. This can be determined by the ammeter, if it is incorporated in the generator. Patients experience no sensation except that of the slight warmth and the smell of ozone during treatment with the mercury arc.

A time clock should always be used to measure the time of exposure. For general irradiation, the body exposures may be divided into quadrated areas. At the end of the treatment, the hood is closed and the lamp is kept burning if there are other treatments to follow. This keeps the intensity of radiation on an equal level and actually prolongs the life of the burner. At the end of treatment, patients are ready to leave the office as soon as they are dressed.

Dosage. The erythemal response of the individual patient serves as a guide for dosage. For general irradiation, the first dose is usually one that causes a minimal erythema. The principal factors in dosage are distance of the burner and duration of exposure. These will vary according to the efficiency of the apparatus, the individual sensitivity of the patient, and the progress of treatment. As patients are irradiated with ultraviolet, they develop an increasing tolerance, enabling them to stand successively larger doses.

Efficiency of Ultraviolet Lamps. Various types of apparatus produce a minimal erythema at various distances and exposure times. The efficiency of one's apparatus—which is chiefly dependent on the condition of the burner in high-pressure mercury lamps—should be checked from time to time by simple skin tests; the same tests also serve to test individual sensitivity of patients.

A simple method for testing is the following: The upper arm is covered by a shield made from a large manila envelope, or by a sleeve made of black cloth, in which five small holes are cut. Under this shield is placed a shutter strip of the same material. The forearm and the face are protected by a towel. The arm is placed at 30 inches directly under the lamp burning at full strength. The shutter strip is withdrawn successively from the openings at intervals of 5 seconds. The exposure is ended 15 seconds after the last hole is uncovered. This results in a progressive period of total exposure for the various openings, ranging from 15 seconds for the fifth opening to 35 seconds for the first. Within a few hours, there should be an erythema visible over one or more of the areas exposed. The exposure time of the area that becomes pale next morning shows a first-degree erythema dose and indicates the average dosage for it at 30 inches. With the weaker lamps, the exposure times would be from 30 seconds to 240 seconds.

In administering dosage, the three principal factors are distance and angle of the burner, duration of exposure, and frequency of irradiation.

Distance from the Burner. It is advisable to start treatment at a standard skin/burner distance of 30 inches and with the exposure time calculated to give a first-degree erythema; on subsequent treatments, one should not change the distance, but gradually increase the exposure time in increments of the minimal erythema dosage. In keeping the distance factor constant, there is less chance of confusion or error. When the maximum time of exposure, say 3 minutes with the high-pressure quartz lamp, has been reached, one can begin to change the skin/burner distance. This can be lowered 2 inches at each successive treatment, until the lamp is at 18 inches. A distance of less than 15 inches is not safe for general irradiation because of the possibility of a heat burn from the infrared emissions of the high-pressure quartz burner. There is also more loss due to the angulation of radiation if the lamp is brought too close to the body.

According to the law of inverse square, moving an object to double the distance from a source of radiation cuts the intensity of radiation to one-quarter; this law does not apply quite strictly to radiation sources that are not a point, but a more extended surface. The following table shows the relative intensity of uniform time exposures given at different distances:

Distance (inches)	40	31	26	22	20	17	14	12	10
Proportionate dose	1	1½	2	2½	3	4	5	7	9

Duration of Exposure. The time necessary to produce a minimal erythema in a patient with average susceptibility at a given distance is different for each type of lamp. With the hospital-size high-pressure quartz lamp, 15 seconds at 30 inches is usually sufficient. The less powerful home-type lamps may require a 15-minute exposure to produce a minimal erythema. They are thus not practical for therapeutic effect in skin conditions such as psoriasis, because of the time required as tolerance develops.

As in succeeding treatments a gradual tolerance to radiation develops, the time of exposure as a rule can be safely increased by 15 seconds each time. For general tonic treatment by the high-pressure quartz lamp in the average patient, the second exposure may be given the next day, and the time of exposure should be 30 seconds; further increase of 15 seconds is made at each successive treatment so that, at the end of 2 weeks with treatments 2 days apart, an exposure of 105 seconds is reached. All these treatments are administered at first at the standard distance of 30 inches.

All dosage and distances mentioned must be subject to modification in accordance with the individual susceptibility and the age of the patient and the condition treated. In cases of severe anemia and debility, it may be advisable never to give more than 10 to 15 *seconds'* daily exposure from the standard distance. With second-degree erythema production, however, one must space treatments carefully so as to avoid too intense reactions in rapid succession.

If the treatment is interrupted at any time and later resumed, the time of exposures must be estimated according to the length of time that has elapsed since the last exposure. It has been estimated that resistance to successive radiation increases to a maximum in about 7 days after treatment, remains the same until about the 20th day, and then rapidly decreases during the next 20 days.

Frequency of Irradiation. No erythema dose should be repeated until the reaction from the previous exposure—if any—has completely subsided. With patients treated in hospitals or at home, daily treatments may be given at first; patients coming to the office may be treated every other day.

A course of twelve treatments administered to ambulatory patients during 4 weeks at a rate of three treatments per week is usually sufficient for general tonic purposes, provided that it is accompanied by satisfactory clinical improvement. After a full course of irradiation, it may be advisable to continue irradiation once or twice a week or to stop altogether.

Individual Sensitivity. Blondes are from 40 to 170 per cent more sensitive than brunettes, and women are 20 per cent more sensitive than men. The minimal dose within toleration is best determined by preliminary skin testing, for if an overdose is given, burns or itching may develop. As a matter of safe routine, it is advisable to administer to children and aged people only one-half, to women about three-quarters, and to blondes and red-haired persons about one-third to one-quarter of the average dose.

People with tanned skins and dark complexions can stand an initial dose larger than the average. People with inborn sensitivity usually know about their poor tolerance of sunlight.

Temporarily increased sensitivity to radiation may occur after any procedures that enhance the circulation of the skin, such as an incandescent-light bath, hot bath, or massage given before irradiation. Alcoholic subjects and patients with long-standing malaria or syphilis may show increased reaction, as may persons sensitized by any of the agents enumerated in this chapter.

Area of Body Exposed. In order to play safe in the occasional instances of unsuspected individual sensitivity, the rule holds to divide the time calculated for a minimal erythema dose between the front and back of the body and then apply further radiation in the same way. In patients in whom for some reason only one surface of the body can be exposed—immobilization in cast, extensive dressings, etc.—one-half of the usual treatment time should be given at first and then carefully increased.

An irritative dose should never be applied except to small areas, whereas a tonic dose should be applied to as much of the body surface as possible.

Different body areas react differently to radiation; those with a thick horny layer are the least sensitive. The most sensitive areas are the face, the chest, the abdomen and the back and sacral region; next come the arms and legs, and least sensitive are the palms of the hands and soles of the feet. Flexor surfaces are generally more sensitive than extensor surfaces.

Group Irradiation. The simultaneous irradiation of small or large groups with ultraviolet is sometimes desirable in schools or other institutions, for prophylactic purposes or to overcome the deficiency of natural sunlight. In patients with ailments, therapeutic irradiation should, of course, always be given individually.

There are two methods of group irradiation: (1) So-called solarium units are available as high-pressure mercury vapor lamps permanently attached to the ceiling. Patients are placed on a circular row of cots, suitably spaced. (2) Several lamps are arranged along the sides of a treatment path or "tunnel" along which the individuals walk or are carried by a conveyor belt; or they may be arranged in the form of a solarium shower. The skin/burner distance of the units is so calculated as to prevent excessive sunburn as the patients are passing along or are standing for a short while. The advantage of the second method is that a much larger number of persons can be irradiated in a given period. The eyes of patients have to be suitably protected for the entire time they are near the ultraviolet source.

Local Irradiation. Local irradiation to a circumscribed area of the skin from the usual types of lamps does not involve any new principle, nor are any additional devices necessary. One may use any type of body lamp by simply covering the area not to be treated and irradiating only the affected part. It is important that such areas be thoroughly cleansed of dead cells, scales, and greasy material, which interferes with penetration. The dosage in local irradiation will depend on the condition to be treated.

CLINICAL USES OF ULTRAVIOLET RADIATION

The clinical use of artificial ultraviolet radiation has greatly decreased in recent years. Because of its special limitations, it cannot be considered an adequate substitute for sunlight. It is rarely needed for specific antirachitic action unless some disease process interferes with oral absorption of vitamin D. Its greatest use is in the treatment of psoriasis and acne.

General Tonic Effect. Mild general irradiation with minimal or suberythema dosage is occasionally employed for nonspecific effect in many chronic diseases, including mental disease.

Chronic Ulcers. Indolent skin ulcers, particularly chronic decubitus ulcers, are often irradiated locally with gradually increasing erythema doses. The effects cannot be considered bactericidal, and comparable results are obtained with luminous infrared radiation. Proper positioning and strict control of hygiene are even more important factors in treatment.

Tuberculosis. The important role of heliotherapy in the treatment of tuberculosis is a thing of the past. In only a few hospitals is it employed at all and then only as an adjunct to specific chemotherapy. Artificial ultraviolet radiation is even less useful and is contraindicated in the presence of active progressive disease.

Skin Conditions. The employment of ultraviolet irradiation, general as well as local, in dermatology has undergone a period of extended reevaluation.

Psoriasis. The combination of crude coal tar ointment and ultraviolet radiation is often one of the most effective methods of treating psoriasis. It is of utmost importance that this form of treatment be used only during the subacute phase. For sake of safety, a test dose of the ointment may be applied to a small area of skin for 24 hours to test for sensitivity reaction. The same may be done with test dosage of ultraviolet to determine a safe minimal erythema. The combined treatment consists of irradiating the entire body, usually in quadrated areas, with a minimal erythema dose through a thin layer of the ointment. Usually, one increases the ultraviolet dosage daily by multiples of the initial dose until a maximum increase is reached, say, in 2 to 4 weeks. The skin must be inspected daily for signs of persistent erythema or symptoms of overdosage such as burning and itching. Dosage is then reduced according to the judgment of the dermatologist or physiatrist in charge. The tar is usually not applied to the face and scalp.

An alternative method employed is to wash off the ointment before ultraviolet irradiation. Adrenocorticoid ointments are applied under occlusive plastic wrap (Saran Wrap) dressings that keep the skin in a hydrated state. Less ultraviolet dosage is usually indicated with this technique.

Occasionally, high-dosage radiation may be given to individual areas

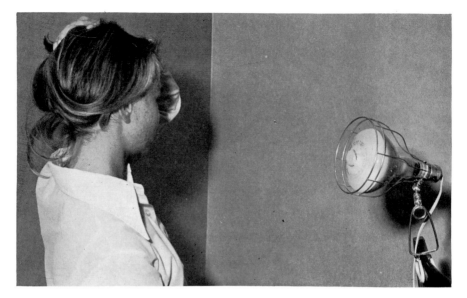

Fig. 7–7.   Ultraviolet home treatment.

of psoriasis in addition to general irradiation. If one area responds well to ultraviolet, all areas respond, even those receiving little radiation.

Acne. Local ultraviolet radiation in the treatment of acne vulgaris is frequently useful in combination with dietary measures and instruction in skin hygiene. Second-degree erythema doses are usually prescribed and repeated as the erythema fades, for example, once a week. Occasionally, blistering doses are prescribed for individual areas with scarring. Even though the effect of ultraviolet radiation is debatable in acne, it remains a popular agent, for acne is generally less severe in the summer. (See Fig. 7–7.)

DANGERS IN ULTRAVIOLET IRRADIATION

The biological action of ultraviolet rays is a photobiochemical reaction following the absorption of rays by living cells, and local chemical reaction develops by irradiation of sterols and proteins. The total number of skin cells irradiated is an important factor in dosage. Dermatitis due to ultraviolet energy ranges from simple erythema to a bullous eruption with pain, chills, fever, and shock. Complications include local ulceration, impetigo, folliculitis, herpes simplex, telangiectasia, and lupus erythematosus. The skin may become sensitized and thereafter react to the slightest exposure. Excessive irradiation of a large area of skin may cause death from general toxemia, but even a weaker dosage applied to a large surface area may cause symptoms and signs of toxemia. Constant strong light when used over a long period of time produces atrophy, wrinkling, and small warty excrescences likely to result in basal or squamous cell carcinoma.

Burns or toxemia in connection with either sunlight or artificial light treatment may occur on account of either hypersensitivity or overdosage or other improper handling of apparatus.

Photosensitivity. There are a few individuals who seem to have an inborn sensitivity to both sunlight and artificial radiation. They may react with severe itching or with rapidly developing dermatitis.

Photosensitization is a condition in which certain drugs or substances present in the system during ultraviolet irradiation cause an increased (photocatalytic) reaction consisting of severe dermatitis. Some of these substances are quinine, trypaflavin, eosin, methylene blue, and other fluorescent dyes. In recent years, interest in the reaction of human skin to ultraviolet light has been renewed, because of the widespread use of certain drugs such as phenothiazine tranquilizers and the tetracycline antibiotics. These drugs alter the cutaneous responses to light. Other drugs are potent photosensitizers and augment the response to light. Ultraviolet is a useful agent in identifying various skin eruptions.

Photosensitization can serve to increase the effectiveness of radiation; this has been done by the indirect administration of fluorescent substances, notably eosin, and by external use of certain substances, notably coal tar (see psoriasis). The sulfonamides have also been described as photosensitizers.

The only way to detect and ward off the dangers of abnormal sensitivity is to administer ultraviolet radiation in all doubtful cases in carefully measured, suberythemal doses.

Overdose. Overdose from any light source may result either from an excessive single exposure or from exposures repeated over too long a period. The immediate visible effect of a single overexposure may be an erythema due to the infrared (heat) rays; exceptionally, there may be immediate blister formation. Ordinarily, the erythema disappears in an hour or so, and in a few hours the effect of the ultraviolet rays begins to show. A dermatitis—skin burn—of varying intensity and extent develops. The longest wavelength that can produce an erythema is about 315 millimicrons. In addition to burns, general symptoms may occur: headache, nausea, high fever, and irregular heart action. Such reactions occurred when patients fell asleep under an ultraviolet lamp or when they insisted upon finding out how much irradiation they could stand. The severe general effects are due to the flooding of the bloodstream with the destroyed protein substances, a severe "protein shock." It is, of course, well known that overdoses of natural sunlight can bring about similar severe reactions.

In the course of ordinary treatments, such severe reactions are very rare, because fortunately a margin of safety as great as 50 per cent exists, and nature reacts much less severely to overdosage from light than to overdosage from roentgen rays. The light-scattering property of human skin provides great protection against actinic damage, with the stratum spinosum scattering the shorter waves most effectively. Melanosomes (melanin granules), in addition to absorbing ultraviolet and visible as well as infrared radiations, bring about considerable scattering.

That eyes may be harmfully affected by ultraviolet is commonly known. Sunlight is ordinarily harmless, but when the ultraviolet component is increased by reflection, it produces "snow blindness." Glowing arcs and metals that emit energy shorter than 295 millimicrons are injurious, and special ultraviolet-absorbing glasses should be worn. The damage usually is limited to conjunctivitis and blepharitis, with prickling pain and uncomfortable foreign-body sensation. Edema, contraction of lids, and corneal erosion may occur. Long exposure to intense ultraviolet rays may produce functional disturbances, such as color scotomas and constriction of the peripheral field. Whether intense ultraviolet rays produce lenticular cataract is still questionable.

Neglecting to protect the eyes against irradiation may result in various degrees of inflammation. Painful conjunctivitis in both patients and careless operators has been reported. A general inflammation of the conjunctiva, cornea, iris, and the lens, known as photo-ophthalmia has been described.

Improper Handling of Apparatus. Improper handling of apparatus usually relates to the home use of ultraviolet. In a fatal accident reported from England, a young man was electrocuted while touching an ultraviolet lamp that he had in a bathroom. It was found that there were about a half dozen ways in which electrical short-circuiting could have happened with that flimsy make of lamp. Of course, the use of any electrical equipment in a bathroom is dangerous.

There is some risk in placing the old-style hot quartz burner directly over the patient because it might suddenly crack. The modern "high-pressure" burner which contains no fluid mercury is free from this danger.

Dangers of Home Treatment.   A survey of the possible ill-effects of self-prescribed and self-administered treatments by the laity was made by a committee of the Medical Society of the County of New York consisting of clinicians, pediatrists, orthopedic surgeons, dermatologists, and physical therapists. There were reported aggravation of cases of quiescent pulmonary tuberculosis; aggravation of various skin conditions, such as eczema, psoriasis, and lupus erythematosus; and numerous instances of burns of varying severity, including dermatitis solaris lasting many months. A number of cases of conjunctivitis were reported, due to careless and unskilled exposure; in children, a decrease of hemoglobin count, when ultraviolet irradiations were continued for a period of months; and some cases of immediate febrile reactions. The committee expressed the practically unanimous opinion of the medical profession that, with so many injurious effects already on record, the prevailing practice of uncontrolled self-treatment by the laity is harmful.

In spite of the vigorous commercial propaganda in favor of home treatment, there are comparatively few instances in which there is real indication for the use of powerful sources of ultraviolet radiation in the patient's home. The danger of overexposure, of careless handling of apparatus and of the indefinite continuation of radiations are all valid reasons against home treatments without the immediate and continuous supervision of a competent physician.

ULTRAVIOLET FOR DIAGNOSIS

The fluorescent effect of "filtered" ultraviolet radiation has found increasing application for diagnostic purposes in recent years. Radiation of about 366 mμ specifically excites intense fluorescence. The interposition of a suitable filter serves to screen out most of the visible light but allows the passage of most of the invisible ultraviolet. All examinations for fluorescence must be made in a darkened room, of course.

In dermatological diagnosis, a Wood's filter—a purple screen of special glass—is employed; this absorbs all visible and short ultraviolet radiation emitted by a suitable short-wave ultraviolet generator and transmits only wavelengths of 390 to 289.2 mμ. When this light is employed in a dark room, all substances with a keratin content, such as fingernails, palms, the weight-bearing areas of the soles and all follicular plugs, appear highly fluorescent, as do any cancerous and precancerous lesions.

According to dermatologists, the most useful application of "Wood's light" is in detection of fungous infection of the scalp. Infected hairs and diseased patches fluoresce brilliantly. This examination also provides a means of determining extent of infection, furnishes a check on progress of the disease or treatment, and is one of the best means of deciding when cure is accomplished. It is an accurate, rapid method for examination of the scalps of large numbers of schoolchildren during an epidemic of ringworm; and pediculosis capitis and pediculosis pubis can also be detected readily. Fading secondary syphilitic eruptions and evolving syphilitic maculopapular eruptions that have not appeared clinically are visible under Wood's light. The true extent of eruption of many chronic dermatoses may be better discerned with this method; cutaneous and mucous membrane lesions that do not show definite color contrast with their background usually can be seen more distinctly. This method has also been used for early detection of x-ray erythema of the skin.

CONTRAINDICATIONS TO ULTRAVIOLET RADIATION

Ultraviolet light is no longer used in chronic debilitating illness. In hyperthyroid subjects and patients with diabetes, severe itching and annoying general symptoms may occur after irradiation; highly nervous people are often made worse and at time show marked pruritus. Menstruation is not a contraindication to irradiation.

All forms of generalized dermatitis as a rule serve as a contraindication to ultraviolet irradiation. In eczema, psoriasis, lupus erythematosus, herpes simplex, erythema solare perstans, xeroderma pigmentosum, freckles, atrophy, keratoses, or prematurely senile skin, irradiation may cause an exacerbation, provoke an attack, or cause other injurious effects.

The possibility of producing cancer in the skin by ultraviolet has been receiving some study in recent years. If the cells of the basal layer of the skin receive an excessive quantity of radiant energy, the two protective processes of cornification and pigmentation become abnormally enhanced (hyperkeratosis and hyperpigmentation), and a third degenerative process starts. Persons lacking in pigment or much exposed to ultraviolet rays show the highest percentage of skin cancer. The developing neoplasm occurs in the place of greatest proliferation, beginning in a wartlike hyperkeratosis, a precancerous change. A cancer develops from a precancerous lesion not only as a result of continuation of the initial insult but from any continued trauma. Thus, ultraviolet rays do not cause cancer in themselves but produce characteristic cell changes leading to precancerous lesions in the skin. Any irritation, including continuously and excessively applied ultraviolet rays, can cause the precancerous change to become malignant. Ultraviolet action spectra may be of some value in the study of carcinoma.

ADDITIONAL READING

American Medical Association: Apparatus Accepted by the Council on Physical Medicine and Rehabilitation. February 1, 1950, p. 101.

Bachem, A.: Special review: Ultraviolet action spectra. Amer. J. Phys. Med., 55:177–190, 1956.

Licht, S. H. (ed.): *Therapeutic Electricity and Ultraviolet Radiation*. 2nd ed. Licht, New Haven, Conn., 1967.

Pathak, M. A., and Epstein, J. H.: Normal and abnormal reactions to light. In T. B. Fitzpatrick *et al.* (ed.), *Dermatology in General Medicine*. McGraw-Hill Book Co., New York, 1971.

Stillwell, G. K.: Ultraviolet therapy. In F. H, Krusen, F. J. Kottke, and P. M. Ellwood, Jr. (ed.), *Handbook of Physical Medicine and Rehabilitation*. W. B. Saunders Co., Philadelphia, 1965.

PART IV

Low-Voltage Electromedical Currents

Chapter 8

ELECTROPHYSICS

The Electron Theory of Matter. Anything that has weight and occupies space is called matter. Matter is composed of over one hundred primary substances known as elements, such as hydrogen, oxygen, mercury, and iron. All complex forms of matter, all minerals, all tissues in animal or vegetable life are formed by the combination of atoms of different elements. An *atom* is the smallest part of an element that can exist. A *molecule* is composed of two or more atoms held in chemical combination. Chemical changes consist of the union, separation, or rearrangement of atoms.

The atoms of all elements are essentially electrical in structure. Each consists of a positively charged nucleus whose mass is practically that of the whole atom. These positive nuclei contain protons and neutrons. Each neutron has a mass of one unit and no charge, whereas each proton has a mass of one unit and a positive charge of one unit. Since only

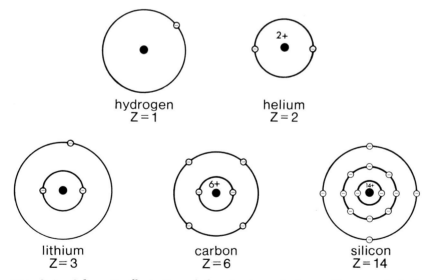

hydrogen
Z = 1

helium
Z = 2

lithium
Z = 3

carbon
Z = 6

silicon
Z = 14

Fig. 8–1. Schematic illustration of the structure of atoms. Every neutral atom contains an equal number of protons ($+$) and electrons ($-$). The nuclei contain neutrons as well as protons (see Fig. 8–2).

the proton has a charge, any given nucleus of atomic number Z and mass number M is now believed to have Z protons and M minus Z neutrons (Figs. 8–1 and 8–2). Surrounding the nucleus in concentric shells are one or more negatively charged particles called *electrons,* whose mass relative to that of the nucleus is negligible. In a neutral atom, the number of protons is equal to the number of orbital electrons. The proton and the neutron are almost equal in weight, and each weighs more than 1,840 times as much as an electron. Since the atoms, unless disturbed in some way, are electrically neutral, the positive charge of the nucleus must be balanced by the total negative charges of its surrounding electrons. By chemical change, atoms may lose or gain electrons, or share them with other atoms.

Experimental investigations have shown that the hydrogen atom is the simplest possible because it is composed of a single proton and a single electron. The atoms of all of the other elements contain more than one proton and more than one electron. In addition, more complex nuclei contain a number of neutrons roughly equal to the number of protons. The unit of atomic weight is that of the lightest of atoms, hydrogen.

Electric Charge. The electron theory is the basis of explanation of electrical phenomena. An object containing a normal balance of electrons and protons shows no electrical properties. If the atomic structure is disturbed by an external force of sufficient strength, such as friction, heat, or chemical action, some of the electrons of the atoms may be driven away. Charging a body consists of taking away or adding electrons. A *negatively* charged body is one that contains *more* electrons than its normal number; a *positively* charged body is one that contains *fewer* electrons than its normal number.

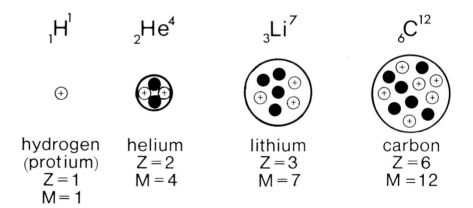

Fig. 8–2. Illustration of the structure of nuclei, showing the numbers of protons and neutrons in several common elements. Carbon has 6 neutrons and 6 protons and an atomic mass of 12. (The atomic number Z is given by the number of protons, and the total of protons and neutrons gives the atomic mass.)

Electrostatics. Frictional or static electricity was the first known form of electricity. The Greeks observed that amber—the Greek name of which is electron—when rubbed, would attract light objects, such as feathers and bits of paper. Gilbert, physician to Queen Elizabeth, discovered that glass, sulfur, resin, and some other substances possessed the same property as amber and he coined the name electricity (electricitas), from the Greek word.

When two dissimilar substances, preferably nonconductors of electricity, are rubbed, one of those bodies may take on an excess of electrons, and the other is left with a corresponding deficit. The one with an excess of electrons is considered to possess a negative charge, while the one deprived of its electrons is considered to be charged positively.

Bodies with the same kind of electricity repel each other, while those charged with different kinds of electricity attract each other. In other words, *like electric charges repel* and *unlike charges attract* (see Fig. 8–3). This is the elementary law of static electricity; it was stated by Coulomb in 1780 that two unlike charges attract each other with a force proportional to the product of their charges and inversely proportional to the square of the distance between them.

Electricity produced by friction is held on an insulated conductor in a state of tension, ready to flow away, and is called "static" electricity, in contrast to "current" electricity, which flows all the time.

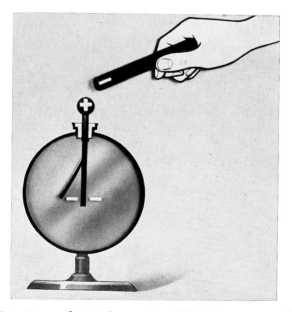

Fig. 8–3. Detecting an electric charge. A gold-leaf electroscope is charged by approaching it with an electrified vulcanite rod. The negative charges are driven toward the leaf, which shows the repulsive effect of the charge.

Table 8–1. Insulators, Semiconductors, and Conductors

Insulators	Partial Conductors	Good Conductors	Semiconductors
Amber	Dry wood	Metals	Germanium
Glass	Paper	Graphite	Silicon
Hard rubber	Alcohol	Watery solution of	Carbon
Paraffin	Tap water	salts, bases, and	
Dry air	Moist air	acids	
Porcelain	Kerosene	Wet wood	
Distilled water			

Conductors, Semiconductors, and Insulators (Table 8–1). Substances that lead off the electric charge quickly are called *conductors;* those that prevent the escape of an electric charge are called nonconductors or *insulators.*

Metals are the best conductors. In all metallic substances, there are always a number of electrons free from their atoms, and as soon as these free electrons are pushed along in the conductor, a flow of electricity will begin. The substances that are good conductors of electricity are also good conductors of heat. Watery solutions of acids, bases, and salts, known as *electrolytes,* also conduct well.

A substance in which there are no free electrons and in which the resistance to the flow of electricity is high is called an *insulator.* To prevent leakage of electricity from the conductors of electric-light wires or from the terminals of electromedical apparatus, insulators are made of glass, porcelain, or hard rubber knobs or plates. There are solid insulators, such as hard rubber, mica, glass, amber, porcelain, and silk, and fluid insulators, such as oils, paraffin, and pure distilled water.

Partial conductors are those substances that, under certain conditions, allow some flow of electricity. Although they offer resistance to the flow of electrons, certain substances, such as germanium, silicon, and carbon, are called *semiconductors.* These substances are used to manufacture diodes, transistors, and resistors for regulating the current in a circuit.

Capacitors. A capacitor is a device for storing electricity; it consists of two conductors placed close to each other but actually separated by some insulating material like glass, mica, or air. An insulating substance that offers great resistance to the passage of electricity by conduction, but through which electrical force may act by induction, is called a *dielectric* substance. In electronic circuits, a capacitor is used to block the flow of direct current while allowing alternating current to pass. It may also be called a condenser, but capacitor is the preferred term in electronic technology.

The Leyden jar (Fig. 8–4) is the earliest form of capacitor; it consists of a wide-mouth glass jar coated by a metal, such as tinfoil, to about two-thirds of its height, on both the inside and the outside. A brass rod extends through an insulated stopper; the lower end of the rod is con-

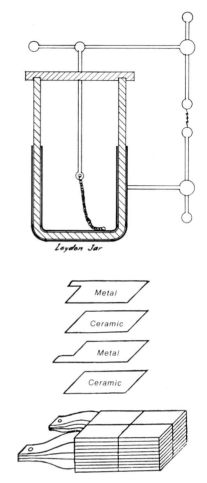

Fig. 8–4. Diagram of Leyden jar and spark gap.

Leyden Jar

Fig. 8–5. Plate capacitor, consisting of alternating layers of metal and ceramic.

nected with the inside coating by means of a brass chain. The rod termi- nates in a knob on its upper end. When the two coats of a charged Ley- den jar are brought into contact, the stored-up electricity discharges itself, usually in the form of an oscillatory discharge, the importance of which will be presented later on. Modern electrical apparatus is usually equipped with plate capacitors, consisting of a number of flat metal sheets separated by insulating material (Fig. 8–5).

CURRENT ELECTRICITY

A stream of loose electrons passing along a conductor is called a cur- rent of electricity. To establish or maintain an electric current, it is necessary that there be a source of energy generating an electric force and that a complete electric circuit be maintained between the higher and lower level of electrons. The path of the current from the generating source through the various conductors back to the generating source is called an *electric circuit.* The electrons move at a certain not very high velocity. The force that makes them move is transmitted at the speed of light. As the electric current flows, the circuit is said to be "closed"; if an interruption or a break occurs, the circuit is said to be "open" and the current ceases to flow

Two forms of current are employed in everyday commercial life, the direct and the alternating. In the case of direct current (D.C.) the flow of electrons continues unchanged in the same direction, while in the case of alternating current (A.C.) the direction of flow changes periodically, as shown diagrammatically in Figures 8–6 and 8–7.

The voltage of the alternating current is represented by a double curve, half above and half below the neutral level. Each part of the curve is called an impulse or alternation, two successive alternations constituting a cycle. The time consumed in the completion of a cycle is called a period. The number of cycles occurring in a second is called the frequency of the current. The ordinary alternating current usually alternates at a rate of 60 per second and is therefore a current of 60 cycles and 120 alternations. In everyday usage, we designate as low-frequency currents those of a frequency of less than 1,000 per second, while the term high-frequency current designates a current with 100,000 or more cycles per second.

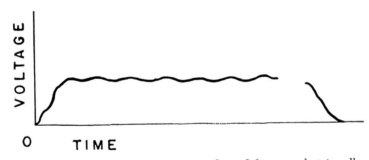

Fig. 8–6.   Diagram of direct current derived from an electric cell.

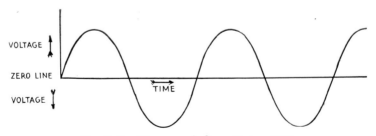

Fig. 8–7.   Diagram of alternating current.

EFFECTS OF CURRENT ELECTRICITY

The existence of an electric current is made evident by the following effects: (1) Heat is developed in all parts of the circuit. (2) Every part of the circuit deflects a magnetic needle brought near it. (3) Chemical action takes place under certain conditions. All forms of currents produce thermal and electromagnetic effects. Chemical action is mainly produced by the direct current; the changes in direction of flow in the alternating current interfere with the regular movement of ions upon which chemical action is based. Currents of very rapid alternation (high-frequency currents) exert no chemical action at all.

Thermal Effects. All electrical currents cause a rise of temperature in a conductor, due to conversion of electricity into heat. The facts regarding this effect was established by Joule in 1877 and are known as *Joule's laws:*

1. The heat produced is directly proportional to the square of the current strength.

2. The heat produced by the same current in different conductors is directly proportional to the resistance of each conductor.

3. The resulting quantity of heat is in direct proportion to the duration of the passage of the current.

Both direct and alternating currents produce heating effects in conductors.

Joule's laws are of great importance in considering the heating action of alternating currents of rapid oscillations (high-frequency currents) on the body. The tissues of the body possess a varying resistance, and those of higher resistance should heat up more when traversed by the electrical current. The electrical current, however, will not pass along a high-resistance path if there is a parallel path of lower resistance available.

The heating effects of electric currents find extended use in everyday industrial life wherever the changing of electric energy into heat or light is desirable. The light of incandescent lamps is produced by the passage of a current through a filament of high resistance, such as carbon or tungsten. A more intense light is made by the carbon arc lamp. In this lamp, an arc is produced by current passing between two carbon rods. In electric radiators and heaters, the resistance of the wire produces the desired heat. In the electric cautery, a loop of platinum wire becomes heated.

The heating effect of electricity on a conductor is directly proportional to the intensity of current and inversely proportional to the cross-sectional area of the conductor; hence the necessity of proper-size wiring in every circuit to prevent overheating of the wires and the consequent danger of fire. The protecting action of an electric fuse is based upon the fact that a current of excess strength develops enough heat in a calibrated length of lead alloy to bring it to immediate melting; thus, the flow of the current is interrupted, and overheating of other parts of the circuit is prevented.

Electromagnetic Effects. A magnet is a substance that has the power to attract particles of iron or steel. It also has the property of setting itself in definite relation to the earth when freely suspended. These effects are produced by the magnetic field surrounding a magnet. There is also a magnetic field around every wire carrying an electric current. An electromagnet consists of a length of insulated wire (electric coil) wound around a soft iron core (Fig. 8–8). When an electric current is passed along the wire, the core temporarily acquires the properties of a magnet.

The electron theory explains electromagnetic phenomena by picturing magnetism itself as due to the movement of electrons within the atom. If a wire carrying a direct current is brought over a magnetic needle and parallel to it, it will deflect the needle at right angles (Fig. 8–9). The magnetic needle points in the direction of the magnetic field. The flow of electrons in the wire makes magnetism. As long as the electrons are kept moving along the wire, the magnetic effect continues. On the principle of electromagnetic influence is based the *galvanometer,* a sensitive instrument for the measurement of direct current; the amount of the deflection of the needle varies with the strength of the current.

Corresponding to the force exerted by a current upon a magnet, there is a reciprocal action of a magnetic field upon a current. If a coil carrying a current is hung in a magnetic field so that it is free to move, it will tend to turn so that its plane will be at right angles to the line of force of the field. This principle finds an important application in the electric motor.

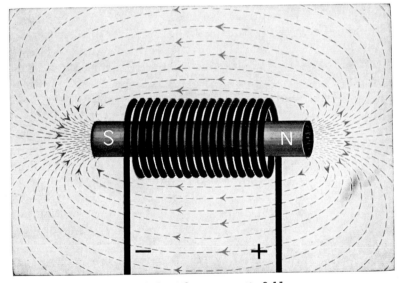

Fig. 8–8. Electromagnetic field.

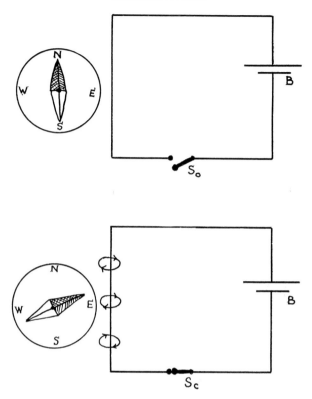

Fig. 8–9.   Deflection of magnetic needle by an electric current.
B, battery; S₀, switch open (no current); S꜀, switch closed (current flowing).

Electromagnetic induction was discovered by Faraday in 1831, who observed that it is possible to "induce" a flow of electricity in a coil of insulated wire if a magnet is moved toward or away from this coil or if the coil is moved toward or away from the magnet. The two most important laws of Faraday are: (1) An alternating electric current is generated ("induced") in an electric circuit whenever in a nearby circuit an electric current of varying strength (an interrupted direct current or an alternating current) flows (Fig. 8–10). (2) An alternating electric current can also be induced in an electric circuit if a magnet is moved near to it or if the circuit is moved in relation to the magnet (Fig. 8–11). In combining both aspects, Faraday's law states that the "electromotive force generated in a conductor is proportional to the rate of change of magnetic flux through the circuit."

Electromagnetic induction also enables us to turn mechanical power directly into electrical power and, through the means of the dynamo, serves as the basis for the large-scale production of electricity. In the most important devices in the modern uses of electricity, such as the

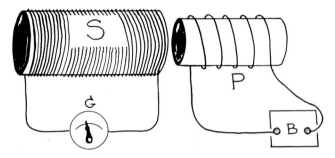

Fig. 8–10. Production of current in a secondary coil by an alternating current flow in a nearby coil. *P*, primary coil; *B*, A.C. source; *S*, secondary coil; *G*, galvanometer.

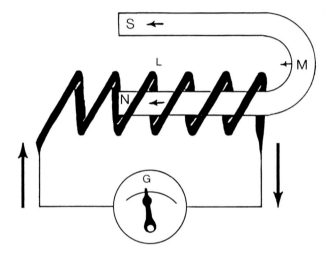

Fig. 8–11. Production of current by movement of magnet surrounded by a coil. *L*, coil; *M*, magnet; *G*, galvanometer. Arrow indicates motion of magnet.

faradic coil, the induction coil, the electric motor, the electric bell, the radio transmitter, the telephone, and the radio receiver, as well as in most electrotherapeutic apparatus, the principle of current production is usually linked up with electromagnetic induction.

Chemical Effects. Solutions of acids, bases, or salts, known as electrolytes, dissociate into free atoms or groups of atoms. These free atoms all bear an electrical charge: bases, metals, and alkaloids are electropositive, acid radicals are electronegative. These electrified particles have been named ions, or wanderers. When a direct electrical current is applied to an electrolytic solution, the ions begin to wander; those with a positive charge are attracted toward the negative pole, or cathode, and those with a negative charge toward the anode, or positive pole. The process of dissociation is known as electrolysis.

The electrical decomposition of an electrolyte is a complicated process. It consists essentially of two phases and is shown in the example of the decomposition of a solution of common salt. (1) Primary reaction: redistribution of ions. (2) Secondary reaction: forming of new chemical bodies at the electrodes (Figs. 8–12 and 8–13).

The chemical effects of the direct or galvanic current are extensively used in industry for electroplating and electrotyping, and also for production of chemicals on a large scale. In silverplating, for instance, the

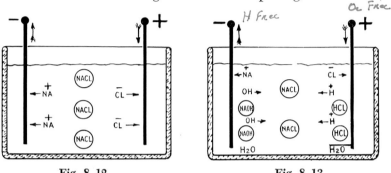

Fig. 8–12   Fig. 8–13

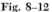

Fig. 8–12. Primary chemical reaction in salt solution under the influence of a direct electrical current. Redistribution of ions in the solution. Sodium ions migrate to cathode, chlorine ions to anode, undivided sodium chloride molecules move in no definite direction.

Fig. 8–13. Secondary chemical reaction in salt solution. Formation of new chemical bodies at the electrodes. Sodium ions become neutralized at the cathode, and caustic soda and free hydrogen are formed ($2Na + 2H_2O = 2NaOH + H_2$). Chlorine ions become neutralized at the anode; hydrochloric acid and free oxygen are formed ($2Cl_2 + 2H_2O = 4HCl + O_2$). At the negative pole, as a rule, bodies of alkaline reaction are formed (litmus turns blue), and at the positive pole, bodies of acid reaction are formed (litmus turns red).

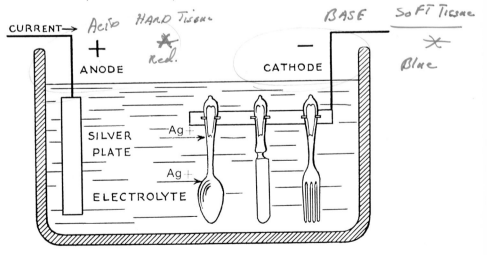

Fig. 8–14. Diagram of silverplating.

article to be plated is immersed in a solution of some silver salt and attached to the negative pole while a rod of silver is used at the positive pole. When the current flows, a thin coating of silver is evenly deposited all over the surface of the object connected to the cathode (Fig. 8–14).

ELECTRICAL UNITS

The analogy of water flow has been employed for a long time to visualize the conditions of the flow of electrons through a conductor. Water will remain stationary in a pipe unless pressure is present to cause it to move. Such pressure is furnished either by a pump or by a difference in level between a high tank and the ground. Similarly, a difference of potential sets up the flow of electrons and is brought about by a generator of electricity. The pressure or tension of the electrical current is in direct proportion to the difference of potential and is known as the electromotive force (emf) or voltage.

Unit of Current: The Ampere. The rate of a current of water flowing through a pipe may be expressed as a certain number of gallons per second. Similarly, the rate of a current of electricity may be expressed as a certain quantity of electricity flowing per second past a certain point (Table 8–2). By international agreement, the quantity of electricity that deposits 0.001118 gram of silver is *one coulomb*, and the current that deposits silver at a rate of 0.001118 gram per second is *one ampere*. The ampere is the unit quantity of electricity flowing per second and serves as the unit of measuring the flow of electricity.

For commercial purposes (lighting, starting motors, etc.), a current flow of several hundred amperes may be used. For electromedical work, a much lower rate of flow is required; therefore, as a measuring unit, only the *milliampere* is employed (1 mA = 0.001 ampere).

Of the various therapeutic currents, the static current employs the smallest rate of flow of electricity, 0.1 to 1 milliampere; the faradic cur-

Table 8–2. Comparison of Water System and Electricity

Water System	Electricity
Pressure or head	Voltage or potential
Rate of flow or volume per unit second	Amperage
Pump	Dynamo or generator
Pipes	Wires or conductors
Water circuit	Electric circuit
Valves	Switches
Valve open (water flows)	Switch closed (current on)
Valve closed (no flow)	Switch open (no current)
Pipes leaking	Short circuit
Pipes stopped up	Open circuit (no current)
Pressure gauge	Voltmeter
Water meter	Ammeter
Water power	Wattage

rent amounts to little over 1 milliampere; the galvanic current varies from 1 to 20 milliamperes; the largest rate of flow is used in high-frequency treatments from 500 to 1500 milliamperes, and more.

Unit of Resistance: The Ohm. A stream of water flowing through a pipe is retarded by the friction of the pipe. A longer and narrow pipe offers more resistance than a short and wide one. The opposition offered by the electrical conductors to the flow of current is known as the electrical resistance, and its factors are the material, the length, and the diameter of the conductors.

The unit of electric resistance is the *ohm,* and by international agreement 1 ohm represents the resistance of a column of pure mercury, 106 cm high and 1 mm^2 in cross section, at a temperature of 0° C, that of melting ice.

Unit of Electromotive Force: The Volt. In order to get water to flow along a pipe, it is necessary to have some driving force—a pump or a difference in water level. In order to get electricity to flow along a wire, we must have an electromotive force. This may be furnished by the difference of potential of an electric cell or battery or by some other electric generator.

The unit of electromotive force or pressure is known as the *volt.* It represents the electromotive force or "push" needed to drive a current of 1 ampere through a resistance of 1 ohm.

The voltage in the commercial current for lighting and power is either 110 or 220. High-power transmission lines carry a voltage from 2000 to over 20,000. The voltage in storm clouds amounts to several millions, bringing about the tremendous electrical discharges of lightning. For a spark discharge across the very high resistance of separated electrical terminals ("spark gaps"), the necessary amount of electromotive force varies with the distance of the terminals. It is estimated that a 1-inch spark requires about 10,000 volts; a 4-inch spark, about 52,000 "effective" volts.

For electromedical currents, the voltage of the supply circuit is considerably modified; it may be decreased by an interposed resistance or increased by "step-up" transformers. Galvanic, faradic, and other tetanizing currents employ up to about 75 volts and are consequently grouped as low-voltage or low-tension currents. High-frequency and static currents employ from several hundred to several thousand volts and are grouped as high-voltage or high-tension currents.

Difference between Amperes and Volts. To understand the distinction between volts and amperes, comparison with water, as shown in Table 8–2, is helpful. With both water and electricity there must be a motive force (head of water or difference of potential) in order to get a flow of current, but we may have the motive force and yet have no current. A closing of a valve in the water pipe acts like an open switch in electricity. There is a motive force or pressure (volts) but no current (amperes). The greater the electromotive force in a given circuit, the greater is the flow of current per unit time; the greater the pumping force or head in case of water, the larger the number of gallons flowing through a given pipe. In other words, electrical current denotes the rate of flow, electrical resistance the opposition that regulates the flow, and voltage the moving force that causes the flow.

Ohm's Law. All calculations of electrical measurements are done with the aid of *Ohm's law*, which states: *In an electrical circuit, the flow of current (amperage) is in direct proportion to the electromotive force (voltage) of the generator and inversely proportional to the resistance of the circuit.*

Ohm's law can be easily explained with the simile of water. When water is forced through a pipe by a pump, the stream that results is in direct proportion to the pressure exerted by the pump and in inverse proportion to the resistance of the pipe. Similarly, in an electrical circuit, the current is directly proportional to the electromotive force or voltage of the generator or electrical cell and inversely proportional to the resistance of the circuit.

On account of the definite relation of these three factors, any two furnish a description of the circuit, since the third can easily be calculated. For instance, the voltage of a simple galvanic cell is about 1.5, and if applied against a body resistance of about 1000 ohms, it will produce, according to Ohm's law, $1.5 \div 1000 = 0.0015$ ampere, or 1.5 milliamperes, of current. So too, if we know that the voltage of a given current is 50 and the milliampere reading when applying it to the body is 10 milliamperes, we learn that the resistance of that part of the body is 5000 ohms.

Ohm's law is of prime importance in every application of electrical current in medicine. Its consideration teaches that there are two ways of increasing the current in a given circuit, either by increasing the voltage or by decreasing the resistance of the circuit through which the current passes. Increasing the size of electrodes, decreasing their distance from each other and decreasing the resistance of the skin by moistening, all tend to decrease the ohmic resistance and thus increase the flow of current through the body.

Unit of Power: The Watt. The work or energy of a flow of water is measured by the number of gallons flowing, multiplied by the pressure in the pipe in a unit of time; similarly, electrical power is equal to the product of the current flowing and the electromotive force (voltage) impressed for a given period of time. A statement that 10 amperes is passing in a circuit or that 100 volts is applied is no complete description of the electrical energy employed. It is necessary to state how many amperes at a certain voltage are passing in a given circuit. The total amount of electrical energy employed in 1 second is the product of volt × ampere, which is expressed in watts.

The *watt* is the unit of electrical power, and 1 watt represents the power delivered when the current flows at the rate of 1 ampere with a pressure of 1 volt. The watt is thus nothing more than the measurement of the rate at which energy is consumed.

The unit of quantity used in figuring the cost of power either produced or consumed is the *kilowatt*. Ten amperes flowing in a circuit where the pressure is 100 volts means power is being delivered at the rate of 1000 watts (10 × 100). One thousand watts are equal to 1 kilowatt, or 1 kW. When power is delivered at the rate of 1 kilowatt for 1 hour, the quantity of power is called 1 kilowatt hour, or 1 kWh. Electric power companies charge a varying amount per kWh, ranging, for instance, from 10 cents in residential districts to 1 or 2 cents to large commercial consumers.

Those installing and employing electrotherapeutic equipment may easily figure out its running cost, as each lamp and each piece of apparatus usually bears a label giving the wattage consumed. For instance, if one operates an electric motor that consumes 250 watts, it will consume 1 kilowatt hour in 4 hours, or ¼ kilowatt hour in 1 hour. If the rate is 10 cents per kilowatt hour, it will cost ¼ of 10 cents, or less than 3 cents to run the motor for 1 hour.

What is the cost of burning a 150-watt lamp for two hours continuously if current cost 10 cents per kilowatt hour? 150 watts multiplied by 2 amounts to 300 watt hours, or less than ⅓ kilowatt hour. Thus the cost would be a little over 3 cents for 2 hours, or about 1½ cents per hour. These calculations show that, after all, the cost of electric power is almost the smallest of the expense items involved in electrotherapy.

Unit of Capacity: The Farad. One farad represents the capacity of a condenser that, when charged with 1 coulomb, gives a difference of potential of 1 volt. This unit is so large that one-millionth of it is taken as the practical unit: The capacity of condensers is usually expressed in *microfarads*.

DEVICES FOR MEASUREMENT AND REGULATION

Instruments for measuring the amperage and voltage of the direct and alternating current are based on the electromagnetic effects of the current. A meter consists of a box having a magnetic device that actuates a pointer in proportion to the current passing through the meter.

Ampere Meters and Voltmeters. An *ammeter* (contracted form of ampere meter) measures the rate of flow of the electric current. Most of the electromedical meters read in milliamperes, expressing 1/1000 of an ampere. Such a meter is called a milliampere meter or, in abbreviated form, a *milliammeter*.

Meters for direct current are constructed on the principle of the galvanometer—which utilizes the electromagnetic deflection of a pointer connected to an electric coil. A permanent magnet maintains a uniform

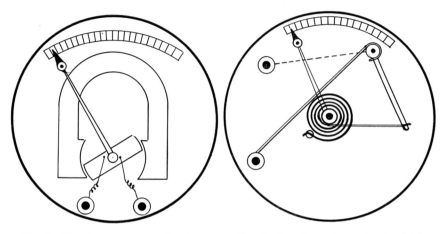

Fig. 8–15. Ampere meter for direct   Fig. 8–16. Hot-wire meter for high-
current.   frequency current.

magnetic field through which the current to be measured flows. A rotating force is exerted upon the coil in proportion to the current strength. The pointer of the meter connected to this coil is deflected accordingly (Fig. 8–15).

Alternating current meters employ a small rectifier to change the alternating current to direct, the meter itself being of the direct current type.

Meters for high-frequency current are designed on two different principles:

(a) Hot-wire type—in which the heating effect of a current causes an expansion of the wire in proportion to the current strength. As the wire is attached to a rotating drum, the movement of the wire causes a deflection of the pointer (Fig. 8–16).

(b) Thermocouple type, based on the principle of the thermocouple. A thermocouple consists of the junction or joint of two dissimilar metals. When such a joint is heated, a difference of potential (emf) is developed that is proportional to the temperature of the junction. The current that flows in a circuit due to the voltage so developed is always a direct current, regardless of the nature of the heating agent. Hence, a high-frequency current forced through a thermocouple will generate heat in the junction, which in turn develops a direct current in proportion to the heat generated by the high-frequency current. By connecting the wires from each side of the thermocouple to the moving coil of a very sensitive direct current meter that has been properly calibrated, readings are obtained in high-frequency milliamperes. Such a meter, referred to either as a high-frequency or a radio-frequency meter of the thermocouple type, is now used in most of the high-frequency apparatus.

A *voltmeter* serves for the exact measuring of the voltage of the electric current. Such measurement is important for more accurate work, for instance in electrodiagnostic procedures (chronaxie measurements). A voltmeter is a sensitive ammeter that has a high resistance of some thousands of ohms placed in series with it so that the current that flows through the meter is extremely small and is a function of the voltage. Thus, with a scale calibrated in volts, it gives a reading directly in volts (Fig. 8–17).

All meters require accurate calibration from the start and must be treated with the greatest of care. The pointer in the better-quality meters revolves in a carefully constructed socket, consisting of some hard precious stone, usually a ruby, that is very sensitive to jolts and vibrations. A meter must likewise be very carefully guarded against strains produced by too strong a current. Most meters are provided with a set-screw for accurate adjustment. With no current flowing through the circuit, the pointer should be checked and carefully adjusted to zero.

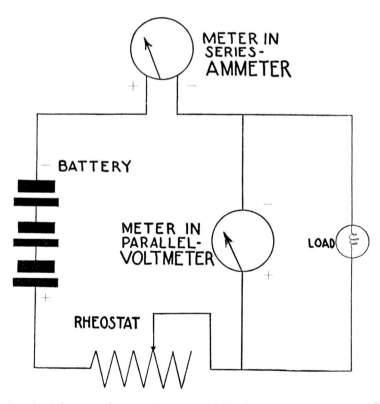

Fig. 8–17. Schematic diagram showing method of connecting ammeter and voltmeter in any circuit. The ammeter is connected "in series" so that the current passes through it, while the voltmeter is connected across the line—in shunt—so that the full voltage is impressed upon it, yet bypassing the current.

4

For measuring small and large currents applied from the same low-voltage apparatus, two-scale *meters* are used that are so constructed that on proper setting of a control, small currents pass directly through the coil of the meter, while heavier currents pass only partly through.

Measuring Power in Alternating Current Circuits. In alternating current circuits, as a result of the continual variations in intensity and periodic changes in direction of flow of an alternating current, as illustrated in Figure 8–7, a *reactance* is encountered in the circuit that causes a "phase displacement" between the current and the voltage. This means that the current and the voltage are actually out of step with each other, with the current either leading or lagging behind the voltage. The reactance and ordinary ohmic resistance of the circuit combine geometrically to produce a new kind of resistance to the flow of current, known as *impedance.* In order to measure power in an alternating current circuit, a wattmeter must be used for measuring the voltage and amperage. A voltmeter and ammeter would give an apparent wattage higher than the true power being consumed.

In average electromedical equipment, such as diathermy, the actual power being consumed and paid for will vary from 50 to 80 per cent of the apparent power. Where electric sterilizers, ordinary incandescent lamps for lighting purposes, radiant light, and heat lamps are used, the apparent watts will be equal to the true watts, as would be the case if direct current were being used. The reason for this is that these latter devices do not have an appreciable inductance and hence do not introduce reactance in the circuit that would cause the current to be displaced.

Rheostats. A rheostat or resistance unit makes use of the resistance of certain conductors or combinations of alloys placed in the path of the incoming current to the apparatus to regulate the amperage. There is usually a negligible flow of current when the full resistance is in the circuit, and as the control is gradually advanced, the resistance is decreased and the current flow is correspondingly increased.

A rheostat of the type most generally used in electromedical apparatus consists of a single layer of resistance wire wound on a straight or a circular form and so arranged that a sliding contact cuts in or out as much of the coil as is necessary to give the required current (Fig. 8–18).

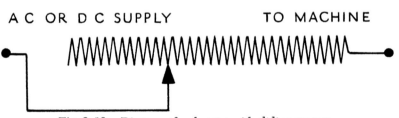

Fig. 8–18.   Diagram of a rheostat with sliding contact.

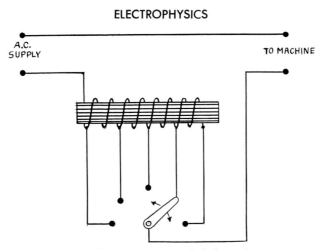

Fig. 8–19.   Diagram of choke coil.

For the regulation of alternating currents supplying electromedical apparatus, a current-controlling device known as a *choke coil* is used. A choke coil consists of several layers of insulated copper wire wound on an open or closed iron core. Taps are brought out from given points of the coil to contact buttons, and a moving contact arm makes connections with each of these and permits the control of current. If a coil of wire forms part of an electrical circuit through which an alternating current is flowing, each alternation induces within the coil a momentary counter electromotive force caused by self-induction. This self-induction is thus used to control the flow of alternating current in a circuit (Fig. 8–19).

A rheostat will regulate the current in both direct and alternating current circuits in the same manner and practically to the same degree, since with both types of circuit, ohmic resistance functions in the same manner. A choke coil will function as such only with alternating current. If used on direct current, it would impede the flow of current only to the extent of its ohmic resistance. The impeding property due to self-induction or inductance would be nil in a direct current circuit.

Chapter 9

GENERATION, CONVERSION, AND DISTRIBUTION OF ELECTRICITY

Thermal, chemical, or mechanical energy can be converted into electrical energy, and this new form of energy can again be readily transformed into heat, light, and other useful forms of energy.

The thermoelectric method of producing electricity is based on the principle of the thermocouple. A series of thermocouples is known as a thermopile or thermoelectric battery, but such a device is employed only for laboratory work. Certain materials will generate a voltage when exposed to the visible rays of the sun. They can be used as solar batteries, like those that were an important source of energy in the first Skylab, launched in 1973. For the production of electricity on an extended scale, only chemical and mechanical means of generation are suitable and will be considered here.

CHEMICAL GENERATION OF ELECTRICITY

Cells and Batteries. The chemical production of electricity is caused by the liberation of electrons when metals go into chemical solution. In a solid metal, the atoms are in neutral condition.

If a plate of zinc and a plate of copper are immersed in dilute sulfuric acid and connected (outside the electrolyte) by wires to a milliammeter, the latter shows that a current is passing. The electron flow is from the zinc to the copper. Inside the solution, particles of zinc enter the solution as positive ions and leave behind two electrons on the zinc plate. The positively charged hydrogen ions are repelled by the zinc ions toward the copper plate, on which they appear as free hydrogen, having picked up an electron from the copper plate. The copper thus becomes positively charged, while the zinc plate becomes negatively charged.

Each of the known metals, when employed in a galvanic cell, produces an electric potential characteristic of that metal. In the *electrochemical series* of metals (and carbon, an exception), any metal is electropositive to any other following it. The series is as follows: carbon, silver, mercury, copper, lead, tin, nickel, iron, aluminum, zinc. The farther apart the metals in the series, the greater potential difference can be obtained.

A *galvanic cell* consists of two metals and an electrolyte. The positive terminal or anode is the binding post at which the current leaves the anode; the negative terminal is the binding post at which the current returns to the cathode. In the copper-zinc cell, the copper plate is the positive and the zinc plate is the negative electrode; in the zinc-carbon cell, the zinc plate is the negative and the carbon the positive electrode. The signs positive or anode (+) and negative or cathode (−), on instrument boards, plugs, and sockets have no other meaning than that of designating the direction of the flow of the current. The current always flows from the higher level to the lower level, *i.e.*, from the anode to the cathode; the electrons themselves flow from the cathode to the anode (Fig. 9–1).

Wet cells are no longer used because of the secondary changes in the substance of the electrolytes and in the electrodes, with a resulting electromotive force opposite to the direction of the original current, known as *polarization*.

Dry cells (Fig. 9–2) consist essentially of a zinc container lined with thin blotting-paper, which serves as the negative electrode, and a carbon rod in the center as the positive electrode; a hygroscopic mass, consisting of ammonium chloride, zinc chloride, manganese dioxide, and granulated carbon, combined with water to form a paste, fills the space between the electrodes. The top of the cells is made watertight with a layer of pitch. Dry cells are clean, are easily portable, and have proved useful for modern commercial purposes where an even flow of a small amount of current is needed, as for transistor radios and pocket flashlights. The voltage of an ordinary dry cell is about 1.5 volts, and the average resistance encountered in the body is about 1000 ohms; hence one cell will produce in the body about 0.0015 amperes.

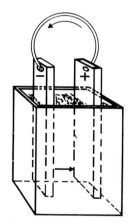

Fig. 9–1. Direction of current flow in an electric or galvanic cell. The electrons flow in the opposite direction.

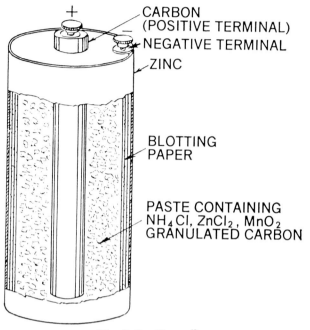

Fig. 9–2. Dry cell.

An *electric battery* consists of a number of cells joined together in series. The *mercury battery* derives its energy through the reaction of mercury oxide and zinc with an electrolyte of potassium hydroxide. Unlike other batteries, the mercury battery tends to have a constant voltage. Besides being extremely small (about three times the size of a dime), it has a voltage of 1.3 volts.

Nickel-cadmium cells are available in button, rectangular, and cylindrical shapes. They are rechargeable by the application of an external electrical source. The nickel-cadmium cells are often used in a series combination for higher voltages.

Storage batteries are "reversible" batteries that can be loaded with electric energy from the line current; almost all the energy thus put into them can be taken out again; this process can be repeated for years without renewing the battery. The metal used in common storage batteries is lead, and the electrolyte is sulfuric acid.

MECHANICAL GENERATION AND CONVERSION OF ELECTRICITY

Dry cells and batteries are somewhat expensive sources for producing large quantities of electricity. Faraday's epoch-making discovery of electromagnetic induction laid the groundwork for the modern age of electricity by making possible the convenient, cheap, and wholesale trans-

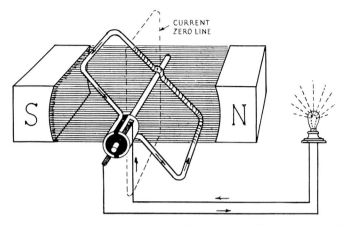

Fig. 9–3. Diagram of generator. In any closed circuit that is penetrated by lines of force of varying intensity, an electric current is induced. This diagram represents a wire loop, rotating in a magnetic field. With every half revolution the number of lines of force by which it is penetrated changes from zero to maximum and back to zero; the intensity of the current generated within the loop and the light from the electric bulb connected to it vary correspondingly.

formation of mechanical energy into electrical energy. Electricity is generated at central stations and from there is distributed through suitably insulated electric wires to homes, offices, and factories.

The Generator. The generator (Fig. 9–3) is an apparatus for the conversion of mechanical energy into electrical power. Its chief parts are (1) the magnetic field, produced by electromagnets or powerful permanent magnets; (2) the armature, a coil of insulated wire mounted around a specially designed iron core; (3) the collecting mechanism which consists of metallic brushes (to make a sliding contact) and slip rings (copper rings that rotate with the armature) in alternating current generators (Fig. 9–4) or a commutator (a split-ring device to collect a direct current) in direct current generators (Fig. 9–3); and (4) an activating mechanical power—steam, gasoline or water power—that keeps either the armature or the electromagnet moving in relation to the other. The mechanical power expended in rotating the armature is transformed into electrical energy, because the rotation sets up a magnetic force that opposes this rotation, and the energy spent to overcome this force becomes the electrical energy.

The Electric Motor. The electric motor is the reverse of the generator, for it is an apparatus for the conversion of electric energy into mechanical energy. It consists of an armature rotating in a magnetic field. The electromagnetic force will tend to rotate the armature, and the shaft of the armature transfers the mechanical power created by this rotation by gearing or belt to other apparatus. Motors are built for operation on

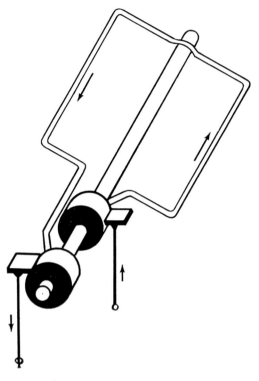

Fig. 9–4. Slip ring in alternating current generator.

either alternating or direct current, and certain small motors may be used on both alternating and direct current.

The Induction Coil.   This is a device for the production of an induced (faradic) current from a direct current source. Its essential parts are (1) a primary coil consisting of a few turns of insulated thick wire wound around a soft iron core, the latter strengthening the magnetic field around the primary coil; (2) a secondary coil, consisting of many turns of insulated fine wire; (3) an automatic circuit interrupter or vibrator that makes and breaks the current in the primary coil (Fig. 9–5). When the switch is closed and a direct current is started through the primary winding (P), the iron core is magnetized and attracts the iron vibrator clapper (CL), which is mounted on a strip of spring steel (SP). The vibrator bends to the right, breaking the primary circuit at the point of the screw (CS). With the current flow stopped, the iron core is demagnetized and the spring of the interrupting device restores contact of the vibrator, thus closing the circuit again ("makes" the current). Each time the circuit is made, the magnetic field grows, inducing a current in the secondary winding in one direction; and each time it is broken, the field falls, inducing an oppositely directed current. Because the early faradic coil

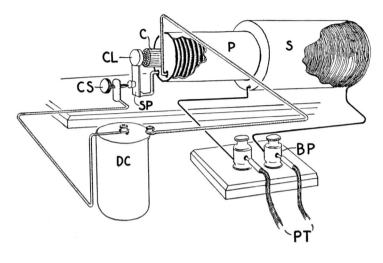

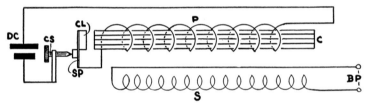

Fig. 9–5.   Diagram of laboratory induction coil (faradic coil). *P*, primary winding of heavy wire turns; *S*, secondary winding of fine wire turns; *C*, soft iron core; *CL*, vibrator clapper; *SP*, spring; *CS*, contact screw; *PT*, leads to patient.

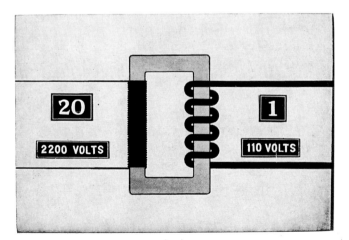

Fig. 9–6.   Diagram of transformer with iron core.

delivered alternating current of brief duration, it was used as a qualitative diagnostic aid in differentiating lower motor neuron disease.

The Transformer. The transformer is a device that changes the voltage in alternating currents. It consists of two coils side by side, having a common "core" of soft iron (Fig. 9–6); one coil has many turns of fine wire and the other has a few turns of coarse wire. When an alternating current is applied to the primary winding, the magnetic field will expand and collapse at the frequency of the applied voltage. As the magnetic field expands, a voltage of the opposite polarity of the primary voltage will be induced in the secondary winding. As the magnetic field of the primary collapses, a voltage of the opposite polarity is induced in the secondary by the change in the direction of the collapsing magnetic field. The frequency of the induced voltage is exactly the same as that of the primary voltage, but the secondary voltage is 180 degrees out of phase with the primary (in the opposite direction). The emf or voltage induced in one coil is directly proportional to the ratio of the number of turns of wire in the coils to each other.

Alternating currents are easily changed from low voltage to high, or *vice versa,* by means of transformers. In the diagram, for instance, it is required to transform 2200 volts down to 110 volts. The fine wire that is connected to the 2200-volt circuit must have 20 times as many turns as the coarse wire coil that is connected to the low-volt circuit. The voltage in the secondary will be then one-twentieth that in the primary. The energy spent in the secondary circuit is equal to that which the transformer takes from the main line, except for a small amount that is lost as heat in the transformer, about 2 or 3 per cent.

There are two kinds of transformers: (1) Step-up transformers, which raise the voltage of the house lighting circuit for use in electrical apparatus, such as high-frequency and roentgen-ray apparatus; in these transformers the secondary coil consists of a correspondingly greater number of turns than the primary coil. (2) Step-down transformers for the reduction of the high-tension alternating current when it reaches the consumer's home, his office, or the factory. In these, the secondary coil has fewer turns. A transformer may also be used in electromedical apparatus to isolate the patient from the power lines and to prevent dangerous shocks if the patient should touch grounded metal objects.

ELECTRIC OSCILLATIONS AND WAVES

When a spring is bent and released, it oscillates back and forth, coming to rest only when its energy is spent. Similarly, when a capacitor, such as a Leyden jar charged with electricity, is discharged through a circuit of small resistance (an air gap or spark gap), the electron discharge takes place in a back-and-forth rush of current from one charged coating to the other until all the energy is spent in sound, heat, light, and electric waves

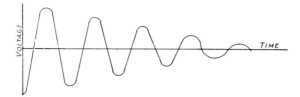

Fig. 9–7. Oscillatory discharge of capacitor.

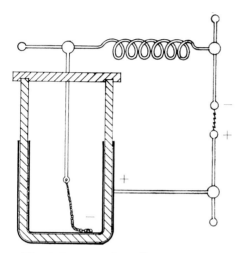

Fig. 9–8. Typical oscillating circuit, consisting of capacitor (Leyden jar), inductance (coil), and spark gap.

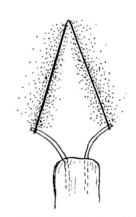

Fig. 9–9. Electron discharge from heated tungsten filament.

(Figs. 9–7 and 9–8). Such a discharge has been shown to consist of a group of sparks rapidly dying out and is known as an *oscillatory discharge*. With the general employment of thermionic devices (see next section), oscillator tubes have largely replaced the use of the spark gap for producing oscillations of various wavelengths. The transistor is now replacing the vacuum tube in many devices.

The oscillations produced by the spark gap or by the oscillating tubes are sustained by the inductance, the most essential part of any oscillating circuit. The *inductance* consists of a solenoid, a coil of copper wire. Such a solenoid offers very little ohmic or "conductive" resistance to the passage of a direct current but offers an enormous "inductive" resistance to the oscillating current that the electrical energy of the condenser or capacitor discharges. Each turn of the solenoid acts as an impedance to the flow of current; as a result, instead of a sudden dying out of the electric charge, the current oscillates back and forth. In the vacuum-tube circuit, these wave trains are "undamped," or all of the same amplitude, because of lack of internal resistance; in the spark-gap circuit, they are "damped," *i.e.*, of decreasing amplitude. If there is too much resistance in the discharge circuit, there are no oscillations, just as a pendulum hung in molasses will sink to its lowest position without swinging.

The energy of an oscillatory discharge traveling through the air will set up similar oscillations in neighboring circuits, provided they are in "resonance," just as a tuning fork will excite strong vibrations in a vibrator that is in tune with it. It was shown that these electric waves travel through the air with the same speed as light, 186,000 miles per second, and form part of the huge field of electromagnetic oscillations. These oscillations differ in their wavelengths, varying from a mile to a few millimeters, depending on the physical constants of the oscillatory circuit. AM and FM broadcasting stations depend on electromagnetic waves set up through a high-tension transformer and sent into the air from an aerial or antenna. Electrical waves produced in the oscillator tube circuit of an electromedical apparatus are conducted through cords or cables to the body as a *high-frequency* current and employed under the name of short-wave diathermy for medical and surgical treatments.

ELECTRONICS

In recent years, the use of vacuum tubes has become quite commonplace and has played an important part in the development of many technical devices. Some of these, such as the radio, radar, television, and similar commercial devices, are well known. Others are of great scientific interest. The cathode ray tube is a vacuum tube electron device that has greatly added to scientific knowledge through visualization of electrical currents. The photoelectric cell has not only been of use to the scientist but is finding increasing commercial application. The thermionic vacuum tube has found increasing use in electromedical apparatus.

Thermionic Emission. Physicists have known for over a hundred years that when a metal is brought to incandescence, the air immediately surrounding it becomes a conductor of electricity (Fig. 9–9). This conductivity is due to the emission or "boiling off" of free electrons from the heated metal. This process is very much like that of the evaporation of water or emission of steam, which is caused by the agitation of the molecules of water overcoming the surface tension. In the ordinary electric incandescent bulb, the "boiled-off" free electrons are drawn back to the filament because when an electron escapes from the metal, the metal is left with a positive charge that attracts the negatively charged electrons. Therefore, there are almost as many electrons falling back into the filament as are "boiled off."

While working on the development of the incandescent lamp in 1882, Edison noticed that when he placed a small metal plate in the lamp, as shown in Figure 9–10, and connected this plate to the positive terminal of a separate battery known as a "B" battery, a sensitive galvanometer would indicate a current flow. When the plate was connected to the nega-

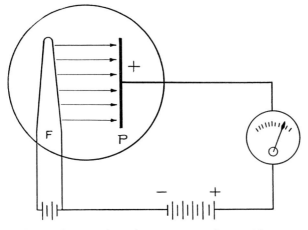

Fig. 9–10. Edison Effect I. When plate is connected to positive potential, electrons flow from filament to plate, as indicated by the swinging out of the needle of the milliammeter.

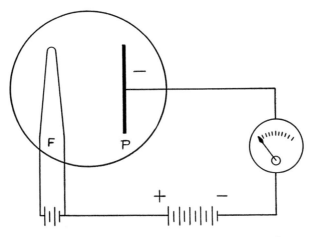

Fig. 9–11. Edison Effect II. When negative charge is given to plate, no electrons will flow in plate to filament circuit.

tive side of the battery, as shown in Figure 9–11, no current would flow. This phenomenon became known to physicists as the "Edison effect." It remained a physical curiosity, but not until the development of the electron theory was it possible to understand the action that took place, which is now known as thermionic emission.

The explanation of the Edison effect is as follows: If a metal plate is inserted into the bulb as shown in Figure 9–10 and is connected to a positive terminal of a direct current source, the free negatively charged electrons swarming about the heated filament source are attracted to this positively charged plate; since a moving stream of electrons constitutes an electric current, there will be a flow of current from the plate to the filament. This can be shown by a galvanometer. If the plate is given a negative charge, as shown in Figure 9–11, no current will flow because the negatively charged plate will repel the electrons emitted from the filament.

Vacuum-Electronic Devices. The discovery of the principle of thermionic emission led to the construction of a large number of thermionic or vacuum-electronic devices. The main feature of each of these is an evacuated glass bulb known as a vacuum tube, and the number and type of metal electrodes contained in it determine its physical characteristics and function.

The *two-electrode tube* or *diode* was developed by Fleming in 1915. It contains a metal filament and a plate. The filament is heated by being connected to a source of current, and a second source of current is connected to the plate and the filament. When an alternating current is applied to the plate, a current will flow from the filament to the plate only while the plate is charged positively, and no current can flow during the negative phase of the A.C. A tube of this kind will conduct current in one direction only, and this action enables the employment of this tube for "rectifying" an alternating current flow, by shutting off every other alternation and changing it into a direct current flow. The vacuum tube acts as a "valve," allowing current to flow in one direction only— from the plate to the filament—and the result is an interrupted, unidirectional, pulsating current flow. Such a tube is known as a *rectifier*. It serves to change the alternating current into a direct current by *vacuum tube rectification*. The rectified current can be "filtered" by suitable inductance and capacitance until it is made into a smooth galvanic current as produced by an electric cell or battery.

The *three-electrode tube* or *triode* contains as a third element a fine wire mesh, known as the grid. The purpose of this is to control the flow of electrons from the filament to the plate. The electrons passing from the filament to the plate must pass through the spaces in the mesh, and

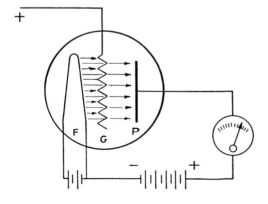

Fig. 9–12. Diagram of functioning of amplifier tube. The third element or grid introduced between the filament and plate of the thermionic tube previously shown in Figure 9–10 serves to influence the current intensity in the plate-filament circuit. A positive potential applied to the grid will increase the plate-filament current as shown by the excursion of the meter.

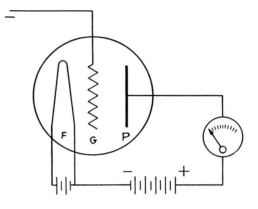

Fig. 9–13. Diagram of functioning of amplifier tube. If the positive potential shown in the previous figure is decreased to zero and then increased on the negative side, the current in the plate-filament circuit will gradually decrease and at a sufficiently high negative potential will be stopped entirely, as evidenced by the lack of excursion of the meter.

their passage to the plate is controlled to any desired extent by varying the voltage applied to this grid. If a positive charge is applied to the grid, as shown in Figure 9–12, it is evident that this positively charged grid will aid the plate in drawing electrons to it. A negative charge on the grid will cause a decrease in the plate current, and if the grid is given sufficiently high negative charge, the plate current can be stopped entirely (Fig. 9–13).

The triode can be used as an *amplifier tube.* From the foregoing it is seen that any variation in the grid potential will be reproduced on a larger scale in the plate circuit. Only a small voltage is needed to obtain changes in the current flowing through the tube. Fluctuations or oscillations of a weak grid potential cause corresponding fluctuations of a much higher amplitude in the anode current through the tube; in other words, the potential impressed upon the grid is amplified in the anode circuit. The control of the current through the tube, and thus through the circuit of which it is a part, is obtained by applying the potential whose characteristics are to be reproduced on an amplified scale to the grid. When used in the manner described above, the three-element tube is functioning as an amplifier. If the voltage applied to the grid becomes more and more positive, the anode current increases up to a maximum value known as the saturation current. All electrons emitted are attracted to the anode, and a further increase of the grid potential makes no change in the voltage or the current.

The triode may also be used as a generator of a very high-frequency current; it is then known as an *oscillator tube.*

Modern Vacuum Tubes. There are hundreds of different kinds of vacuum tubes in use today. Some tubes have two electrodes, while others may have as many as seven (pentagrid converter with five grids). An important development of the modern tube is the employment of an indirectly-heated cathode in place of a filament as a source of thermal electrons. A fine tungsten wire filament is threaded through two small holes of a porcelain-like insulating rod. Fitting snugly around this rod is the cathode, a metal cylinder coated on the outside with a thin layer of thorium, strontium, or cesium oxide. These particular oxides provide a copious emission of electrons when heated to a dull red.

Gas-Filled Electronic Devices. An electrical current of high voltage passing between two electrodes in a glass tube filled with gas at low pressure causes a glow discharge to take place. This is due to ionization, or breaking up of atoms of the gas and the freeing of a stream of conducting electrons. This differs from thermionic emission of electrons from a heated wire in a vacuum tube. Various colors are produced in the vacuum between the electrodes, depending on the gases ionized: In a neon-filled tube, the glow discharge is reddish; mercury vapor gives a bluish color; and so on. When direct current is used to energize the tube, the ionization is brightest near the cathode (negative electrode); when alternating current is used, both electrodes are equally bright. Mercury vapor tubes used in therapeutic machines for rectification show a glow discharge.

Two-electrode vacuum tubes (diodes consisting of a heated filament and a metal plate) containing mercury vapor at low pressure are extensively used as *mercury-vapor rectifiers,* just like thermionic vacuum tube rectifiers: When the plate is negative, no electrons are drawn from the cathode and no current flows; only when the plate is positive does the current flow. In electromedical apparatus, mercury vapor rectifiers are used in short-wave diathermy machines to convert alternating current from the mains to direct current.

Three-electrode vacuum tubes (triodes) filled with gas are known as *thyratrons.* The larger thyratron tubes contain mercury vapor gas, the smaller ones argon. The tube is usually connected across a capacitor with a charging current. While the capacitor is absorbing the charging current, the thyratron remains nonconducting, but as the capacitor becomes charged, the gas in the thyratron becomes ionized by the rising voltage. When this happens, the tube becomes conducting and short-circuits the capacitor. When the capacitor loses its charge, the voltage drops and becomes too low to maintain the thyratron in an ionized state, so that the tube becomes nonconducting again and the capacitor starts to charge once more. This cycle continues, with production of the wave shape shown in Figure 9–14. The relatively slow rise represents the charging capacitor; the sudden sharp drop, the discharge of the capacitor by the

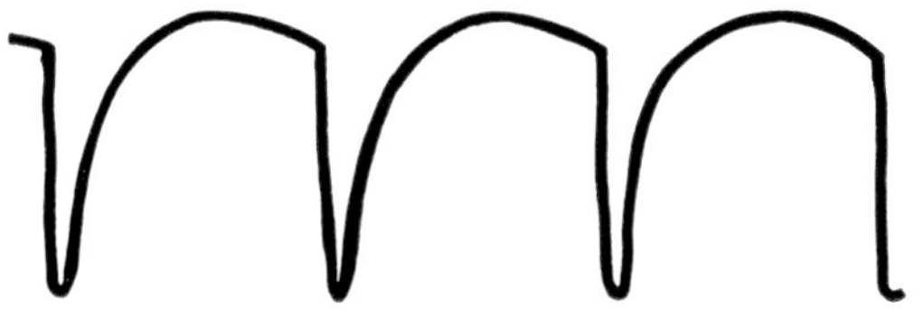

Fig. 9–14. Wave shape of current produced in thyratron tube.

ionized thyratron tube. When the charging voltage is held constant, the rate of oscillation is determined by the size of the capacitor. By construction of a unit so that any one of a number of capacitors may be introduced into the system as desired, low-voltage currents of any desired frequency may be obtained. Extremely simple to control, such currents have perfectly regular wave form.

Semiconductors and Transistors. The field of electronics has made many advances, chief among which is the development of the transistor. Originally, transistors had replaced the vacuum tubes in portable equipment, radios, televisions, and medical equipment such as cardiac pacemaker and stimulator. Today, "solid state" describes the electrical circuitry of the modern tubeless apparatus.

Solid-state physics is a field of research concerned with the study of the physical properties of solids and includes such subjects as the detailed configuration of atoms in solids, the behavior of free and bound electrons in a crystal lattice, the electrical conductivity of both pure substances and those containing impurities, and the magnetic response of solids at low and high temperatures.

Semiconductors are certain solids that are neither good conductors nor good insulators. Certain semiconductors are elements listed in the fourth column of the Periodic Table with four valence electrons (electrons in the outermost orbit) (Fig. 8–1), substances such as silicon and

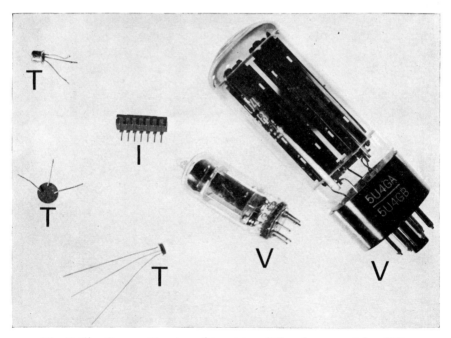

Fig. 9–15. Comparative sizes of transistors (*T*) and vacuum tubes (*V*). *I*, integrated circuit.

germanium. A junction between two different semiconductors may readily permit a current flow in one direction but oppose flow in the other direction. These substances are inexpensively prepared into crystals with impurities (doped), and a small solid pellet is now able to replace various diode vacuum tubes. Both the vacuum tube diode and the semiconductor diode are used as rectifiers.

The *transistor* (Fig. 9–15) is an electronic device that can perform many of the functions of triode vacuum tubes. Besides being extremely tiny, they require little power, in contrast to vacuum tubes. Vacuum tubes fail easily, due to low emission, breakage of glass envelope, and breakage of filaments, whereas a transistor seldom requires replacement. The mechanical and chemical construction of the transistor is so simple that its life under normal application is almost unlimited. The maintenance of transistorized equipment ("solid state") is greatly simplified. Many of the components are so inexpensive that they are considered expendable and "throw-away" items (Fig. 9–15).

A transistor is a current-controlling device that changes its output impedance when the input current changes. They are used as amplifiers and oscillators to improve high-frequency operation. They are used to trigger circuits and to control sweep circuits and timing devices.

A transistor contains three semiconductor elements, while a diode is composed of two semiconductor elements. They do not need time to warm up, nor do they get hot after hours of continuous use. Certain electrical limitations of transistors prevent their substitution in all vacuum tube functions. Diodes and transistors are used in portable stimulators and electromyographs. (Figure 9–16 shows the most common electrical symbols.)

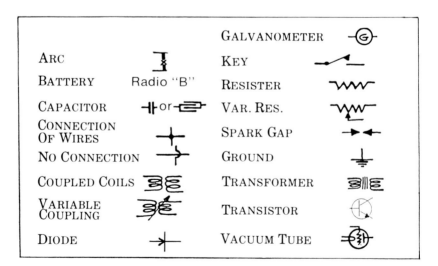

		GALVANOMETER	
ARC		KEY	
BATTERY	Radio "B"	RESISTER	
CAPACITOR	or	VAR. RES.	
CONNECTION OF WIRES		SPARK GAP	
NO CONNECTION		GROUND	
COUPLED COILS		TRANSFORMER	
VARIABLE COUPLING		TRANSISTOR	
DIODE		VACUUM TUBE	

Fig. 9–16. Electrical symbols most frequently employed.

ELECTRICAL CURRENT SUPPLY IN HOUSES AND OFFICES

While the two forms of electric current—alternating and direct—were at one time supplied by central power and light stations, alternating current is now supplied almost exclusively. Alternating current may be changed expeditiously to direct current with electronic rectifiers when unidirectional currents are desired. By generating alternating currents at high voltages (up to 200,000 volts), electrical energy can be transmitted over long distances without much loss in transmission, and at any point along the line the high-tension current can be reduced by a step-down transformer to a low-tension current (220 to 110 volts) ready for general use.

Measuring and Protecting the House Supply. When the current from the mains enters a building, it first passes through a service switch that permits the entire house to be disconnected from the mains. This switch is fused to protect the house circuits from excessive current flow. From the service switch, the current flows through a watt-hour meter where the electrical energy consumption is recorded. The current now passes through the individual circuit fuses or circuit breakers to the various outlets and receptacles.

The Role of Fuses. A fuse is a current-limiting device, consisting of a piece of alloy of low melting point and of a thickness and length calibrated to stand just a certain amount of current. If more than the contemplated amount of current is drawn, the wire rapidly heats up and melts, the fuse blows, and the flow of current is interrupted, thus preventing overheating of electric wires or sparking and the consequent danger of a fire.

Fuses will blow most frequently due to overloading or to a short circuit. Overloading occurs when more current is drawn than is allowed a given circuit. For instance, if a branch circuit is wired and fused for 15 amperes at 100 volts and one turns on a 1000-watt bulb drawing 10 amperes and then tries to light an ultraviolet generator drawing about 9 amperes on the same circuit, one is usually reminded, to the tune of a blown fuse, that the limit allowed has been exceeded. Needless to say, replacing the 15-ampere fuse by a 25-ampere fuse does not solve the problem, as the capacity of the fuse and the wiring in a given circuit are related, and by attempting to draw more current, one overheats the entire wiring and courts trouble and danger, possibly in some inaccessible part of the circuit. To prevent overloading the number of outlets and the wiring in a given circuit, therefore, one must never use a fuse larger in capacity than the maximum safe current.

Short circuits occur if somewhere in a circuit two uninsulated wires come into unexpected contact, as will happen when the insulation in a conducting cord is worn away or one wire in an attachment plug becomes loose and touches the opposite one. This causes an arcing of the current across the short path; on account of the lessened resistance, more current is drawn and, consequently, the fuse blows. A short circuit is by far the most frequent cause of blowing of fuses in the physician's office. Its prevention lies in inspecting all contact parts subject to friction and strain, either at stated periods or whenever they show wear. If a fuse has blown, before replacing it, one should disconnect the piece of equipment in which the short circuit has occurred; otherwise, the fuse will blow again. The hissing noise, sparks, and heat accompanying a short circuit usually make its location easy.

Finally, fuses may blow at times without apparent reason, due perhaps to wear of equipment or to defective construction. In such instances, they simply have to be replaced. Fuses are sometimes made part of electrical apparatus, in order to protect delicate lamps and measuring devices against any excess of current.

Locating Trouble. In order to be able to act at once in case of trouble with fuse, other electrical trouble, anyone employing electricity for therapeutic purposes should know the location of the fuses for each circuit and also on the apparatus itself so as to be able to replace them *after* the cause of the trouble has been found and eliminated. It is advisable that a panel box with all fuses pertaining to the equipment be located in or near the office at a place easily accessible and well lighted. A complete diagram affixed to the inner door of the fuse box should show the outlets covered by each of the fuses and thus make quick repair possible. It is also advisable to have the lighting circuit of the office separate from the therapeutic circuit, so that in case of trouble the lights would not be disturbed, the light sockets then even serving as an emergency supply socket for the apparatus. A sufficient supply of fuses of appropriate size should always be kept on hand in the fuse supply box, along with an electric flashlight in working order, or a piece of candle and matches.

If more than one circuit has failed in the house, as, for instance, a number of pieces of apparatus and the lights on several floors, this usually indicates that one of the main fuses in the meter box has blown or that the trouble may be in the meter or in the supply line outside of the house. In such a case, the help of the electric power company should be enlisted.

In recent years, thermal-operated circuit breakers (cutouts) are replacing fuses. The advantage of this device is that it need only be reset after it has operated and after the cause of the overload has been corrected. Magnetic circuit breakers are also favored in some installations.

Current Outlets. For the efficient working of electrotherapeutic equipment, the proper number and placing of current outlets is both a convenience and a necessity. Starting from the fuse box, each electrical circuit in the home or office includes several outlets either as base plugs or as wall receptacles. A temporary connection to any electric light socket may be permissible for small apparatus, provided that the outlet is wired and fused for the amperage of the particular apparatus. For permanent connections, special outlets, preferably independent of the lighting circuit, are advisable. These should be placed about 3 to 4 feet above the floor so as to be readily accessible for attachment of the connecting line to the apparatus. The number of outlets should correspond to the number of pieces of equipment; frequent plugging in and out causes unnecessary wear and tear on the connections.

Three-element receptables and plugs are desirable, the third element being a good ground connection. Adequate grounding is essential to prevent electrocution and burns, to prevent interference with recording instruments, and most important, to prevent malfunction of cardiac monitors.

ADDITIONAL READING

Becker, C. M., Malhotra, I. V., and Hedley-White, J.: The distribution of radio frequency currents and burns. Anesthesiology 38:106–123, 1973.

Brite, R. J.: *Transistor Fundamentals.* Vol. 1. Howard W. Sams and Co., Indianapolis, 1972.

Upton, M.: *Inside Electronics.* Signet, New York, 1964.

Chapter 10

CURRENTS, APPARATUS, AND ACCESSORIES

General Considerations. Practically all electromedical currents are derived from the commercial lighting circuit. The galvanic current may be drawn *directly* from dry cells or radio batteries. All other currents are obtained from the alternating (A.C.) street current by suitable modification, through transformers and other electromagnetic or thermionic devices.

The source and means of production of any current has no relation to the response of the tissues of the body. The final form of the electrical energy, the technique of application, and the individual condition of the subject will determine the effect that it will exert.

The transformation of the basic electrical energy into the different therapeutic currents is best visualized through the simile of a water system (Table 10–1). Water can be applied either at high pressure or at low pressure, at a large rate of flow or in a fine spray, running continuously or in abrupt squirts or waves. Similarly, the flow of electrons may be even, or interrupted, or reversed, frequently or infrequently, symmetrically or asymmetrically; the rate at which the current is increased from zero to maximum may be slow or rapid, and it may remain at low tension or rise to very high tension.

CLASSIFICATION OF CURRENTS

In classifying electromedical currents, their primary characteristics as well as their biophysical effects are taken into consideration (Tables 10–2 and 10–3).

Table 10–1. *Comparison of Water System and Electric Currents*

Water System	Electric Current
Low pressure	Low tension galvanic
High pressure	High tension
Fine stream	Low amperage
Large volume	Large amperage
Continuous flow	Galvanic (direct) current
Squirts or waves	Interrupted and surging currents

Table 10–2. *Electromedical Currents I—Physics*

Physical Characteristics

Current	Mode of Flow	Approx. Frequency	Voltage	Amperage	Physical Effect
Direct (galvanic)	Unidirectional constant	. . .	Low	Medium	Chemical
Interrupted direct	Unidirectional shock	Manual control	Low	Medium	
Slow repetitive	Unidirectional square waves about 50 msec	5 to 20 per sec	Low	Medium	
Alternating	Sine wave	60 cycle	Low	Medium	Electro-kinetic
Fast repetitive (tetanizing)	Unidirectional square waves 0.5 to 5 msec	50 to 200 per sec	Low	Medium	
Faradic	Rapid asymmetric alternating surges	About 100 per sec	Medium	Low	
Short-wave diathermy	Extremely rapid oscillations	10,000,000 per sec	High	High	Thermal

Table 10–3. *Electromedical Currents II—Principal Forms of Application*

The direct or galvanic current
    Medical galvanism
    Ion transfer
    Surgical galvanism (electrolysis)

Currents of low tension and low frequency
    The interrupted direct current (manual)
    The faradic current (nearly obsolete, laboratory)
    The repetitive square waves
    The alternating current (60 cycles)

High-frequency currents
    Long-wave diathermy (surgery only)
    Short-wave diathermy
    Microwave diathermy
    Electrosurgery: desiccation, coagulation, and cutting

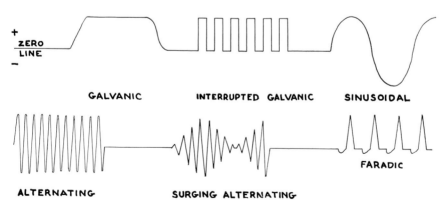

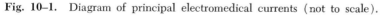

Fig. 10–1. Diagram of principal electromedical currents (not to scale).

The physical characteristics of electromedical currents are direction of flow and frequency of alternation or repetition, voltage or strength, and amperage or volume of flow. The following groupings can be made on the basis of these:

Direction and Frequency of Flow. *Unidirectional currents* are those that flow in one direction without reversal of polarity; the direct current, the interrupted direct current and repetitive square or rectangular waves are unidirectional currents. *Alternating currents* are those that reverse their direction of flow; this group includes (*a*) *low-frequency currents,* with an alternation not exceeding several hundred per second (the faradic and the alternating current belong to this group); and (*b*) *high-frequency currents,* with alternations or oscillations over 1,000,000 per second (long- and short-wave and microwave diathermy belong to this group). Long-wave methods are rarely used today.

Voltage or Tension. *Low-tension* currents are those with a voltage of 100 and less; the direct and the low-frequency currents belong to this group; *high-tension* currents are those with a voltage of several hundred or higher; high-frequency currents involve such voltages.

Amperage or Volume. Since no high amperage or current volume is possible without a corresponding high voltage to produce it, high-voltage currents are, generally speaking, currents of high amperage, employing from 500 to 2000 or more milliamperes, while currents of low tension are currents of low amperage, employing from 1 to 30 milliamperes.

According to biophysical effects, electromedical currents can be divided into two large groups: (1) currents causing ionic changes in the tissues and a minimum of thermal effects and (2) currents causing only thermal changes. The direct and low-frequency currents belong in the first group, high-frequency current in the second. Table 10–3 shows the generally accepted grouping of electromedical currents and their principal forms of application. All these will be fully discussed in their respective chapters.

ELECTROMEDICAL APPARATUS

Some physicians, like some laymen, look upon apparatus either as something mysterious, able to perform curative feats at the turn of a knob, or else they think it is all make-believe. As a matter of fact, all apparatus can do is to deliver a definite form and amount of physical energy to a given part of the body. It is up to the physician to know what physiological effects to expect from such an application and when to make use of it in treating disease and injury. The physician should be able to visualize at all times: (1) the physical events inside the apparatus when the current is turned on from the source of electric power and (2) the physical and physiological changes in the body when the current is applied through the electrodes.

Typical Features of Apparatus. Electrical apparatus for treatment purposes usually consists of a box or cabinet, which contains the electrical unit (transformer, vacuum tubes, transistors, etc.) that changes the supply of alternating lighting current into one of the electromedical currents. Some pieces of apparatus contain dry cells or batteries and are independent of any outside current supply source. All terminals are mounted on insulating material, such as hard rubber or porcelain.

The typical features of the average apparatus are: (1) A *current input* where the cable bringing the supply current from a wall receptacle is inserted. (2) A *main switch* by which the flow of supply current is turned on or off. (3) A *rheostat* or regulator that regulates the strength of the outgoing current and enables the drawing of as much current as needed for the individual treatment. (4) A *milliammeter*—or simply meter—showing the amount of current passing. (5) *Terminals* or current outlets for the insertion of cables or conducting cords that lead the current to the patient. (6) A *pilot* light, which lights up as soon as the main switch is turned on and the supply current enters the apparatus. (7) A *timing device* (time clock) by which the duration of current flow can be set from a few minutes to an hour; at the end of this period, the current is automatically cut off.

CONDUCTING CORDS AND CABLES

The electrical energy from electromedical apparatus is conveyed to the patient by means of conducting cords, or cables, consisting of flexible copper wire surrounded by a suitable rubber or plastic insulation. The thickness of insulation depends upon whether a current of low or high voltage is carried by the conductor.

Conducting cords (Fig. 10–2) used in present-day equipment are, as a rule, of uniform color and serve for the conduction of low-tension

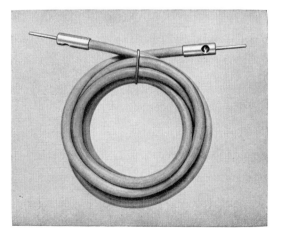

Fig. 10–2. Conducting cord.

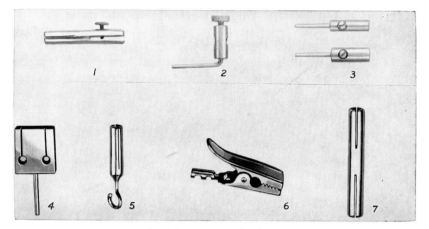

Fig. 10–3. Connectors and cord tips. *1*, single flat connector for cord tip; *2*, bent connector for binding post on apparatus; *3*, cord tips; *4*, double connector for binding post; *5*, hook connector for vacuum or condenser electrode; *6*, spring connector; *7*, double connector to lengthen cords.

(direct and tetanizing) currents. Special cables serve for short-wave diathermy, microwave diathermy, and ultrasound. For galvanic treatment, sometimes cords with different colored insulating covers are employed so as to remind the operator of the different polarities. Conducting cords must be fastened securely at one end to the binding post of the apparatus, usually through a binding screw, and at the other end to the electrode, usually through some clip arrangement.

For fastening conducting cords to the back of the metal electrodes, *clips* or flexible connectors serve (Fig. 10–3). In low-tension moist-pad electrodes, a connection for the conducting cord is usually soldered onto the metal back, and the cord tip is held there by a spring. All such connections are subject to electrolytic deterioration and breaking and should be inspected from time to time. Loose-fitting clips may pull out easily, causing an excess density of current on the skin and an instantaneous burn if they should touch the bare skin.

Cords may get out of order by a break of the copper wire inside the cord's insulation or by a loosening or slipping of the contact between the wire and metal tip. To prove that the current goes through a cord, one may connect both terminals of an apparatus by the cord and turn on a very small amount of current. If the wire is intact and conduction is present, the meter will register at once (be careful not to strain meter by sudden heavy current). Loose contact between the wire and the cord tip is remedied by scraping off the insulation at the end of the cord and reapplying the copper wire by tightening it with the binding screw. To prevent loosening at the cord tips, cords should never be jerked out of the sockets but pulled out gently by holding on to their tips.

Conducting cables for short-wave diathermy consist of heavy insulated cable containing the conducting wires. Microwave diathermy and ultrasound are conducted by coaxial cables. When they are in contact with or close to a good conductor (metal frame of bed or chair), or when crossing each other, they may concentrate some of the electrical energy; such energy leakage heats up the rubber insulation of the cable and may cause it to burst into flame. The most vulnerable part of the cable-pad electrode assembly is the corner where the cable joins; with careless handling, the rubber insulation may crack there and lead to leakage of current and subsequent overheating. Regular inspection of such accessories is, therefore, essential.

ELECTRODES

An *electrode* is a medium intervening between an electric cord or cable and the body. It should consist of a good conducting material whose shape and form can be well adapted to the skin or the cavity.

Water containing some salt is the simplest electrode material and makes perfect contact with an extremity immersed in it. The water bath as an electrode is used for some galvanic treatments. For the great variety of electric treatments, however, most of the electrodes consist of flexible metal plates, either applied directly to the body or separated by moist padding or rubber insulation. Glass vacuum electrodes are used less frequently in high-frequency treatments.

Contact metal electrodes are cut to suitable size and shape from electrode foil—an alloy of lead, tin, and zinc (Fig. 10–4). Metal electrode material comes in three grades of thickness and is sold in rolls by the pound. It is cut by shears into suitable sizes, and it is advisable to leave a small tongue, about 1 by ½ inch, to one side; folded back against the rest of the plate, this tongue serves for attaching the conducting cord (Fig. 10–5). Before use, the electrodes should be smoothed by a light roller like

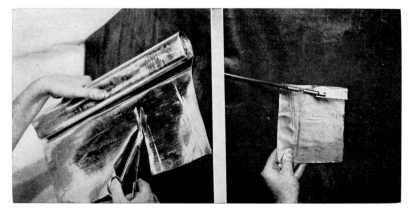

Fig. 10–4.   Cutting electrode foil.   **Fig. 10–5.**   Plate electrode ready for use.

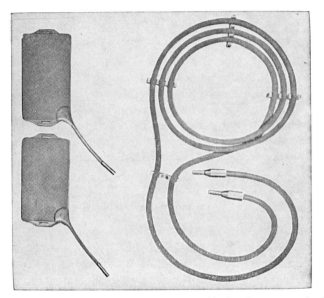

Fig. 10–6. Condenser pads and inductance cable for short-wave diathermy.

those used for photographic prints. They should be cleansed from time to time with soap and water. Plain metal electrodes are chiefly used for iontophoresis. For this purpose, it may be convenient to cover the metal with fabric that can easily be kept moist.

Spaced metal electrodes [condenser pads (Fig. 10–6) and cuffs] consist of flexible metal enclosed in insulating rubber sheath. They are applied to the skin with an interposition of toweling or felt and additional moisture-absorbing blotting or tissue paper. Spaced plates (Fig. 16–1) consist of metal discs enclosed in hard circular rubber treatment drums. They are held at a suitable distance and positioned by adjustable arms. All these electrodes carry a fixed cable connection in one corner and serve for short-wave diathermy treatment.

Inductance cables are single electrodes used for short-wave diathermy with the electromagnetic field technique. They contain a flexible wire surrounded by heavy insulation. They are applied in the form of circular loops around the body or an extremity and also in the form of a "pancake" coil or a treatment drum (Fig. 10–7). Their two ends carry plugs to fit into the current outlets of the apparatus.

Moist-pad electrodes consist of flexible metal plates covered on one side with a layer of soft rubber and bearing a suitable opening for the attachment of the conducting cord. On the side to be applied to the skin, there is a pad of absorbent material of suitable thickness and strength, and this is covered with linen and fastened to the metal plate in back (Fig. 10–8).

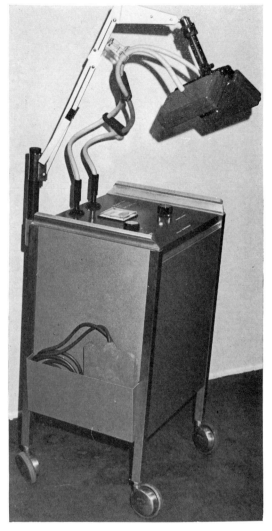

Fig. 10–7. Short-wave diathermy apparatus with treatment drum. (Courtesy of Burdick Corporation.)

Moist-pad electrodes serve for galvanic and low-frequency treatments in which it is necessary to soften the horny layer of the skin for the passage of the current. The covering of the pad electrodes is soaked with tap water or a 2 per cent saline solution. The moist pad also absorbs the acid or alkaline products of the electrical decomposition of the metal and thus prevents chemical burns. The ordinary one-piece pad electrodes can be easily cleansed by soap and water and laid out to dry until the next use. A simple method to provide a clean surface at each treatment is to cover the pad with a fresh layer of loose sterile gauze.

Instead of ready-made moist-pad electrodes, electrode pads of any desired size for galvanic treatments can also be improved by folded hand

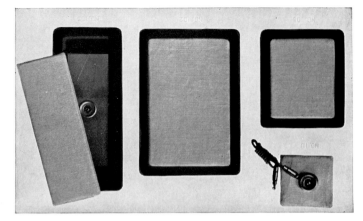

Fig. 10–8. Pad electrodes for low-tension currents. The removable pad allows better cleansing. (Courtesy of Burdick Corporation.)

towels, turkish towels or gauze. In such cases, care must be taken that the material used is of adequate thickness and is thoroughly soaked in saline solution, that it is well folded, and that the metal foil laid on top of it nowhere comes in contact with the skin; also, the conducting cord should be well fastened to it by a clip and safely held there.

Glass electrodes serve for the application of some forms of high-voltage (high-frequency) treatments to the body. *Vacuum electrodes* consist of a hollow glass tube from which the air has been exhausted to a varying degree. Glass electrodes are mounted on an insulating handle to prevent the leakage of current through the operator's fingers.

Securing Electrodes. Electrodes have to be applied and held snugly. Under the back and the chest, the weight of the patient's body will hold the electrodes, while over the thigh, abdomen, and chest, a small sandbag and pillow can be utilized to hold the electrodes with the patient supine. In applying electrodes over an extremity, the face, or other rounded portion, a few turns of a woven elastic bandage, 2 inches wide, will insure an even contact. In bandaging moist-pad electrodes it may be advisable to interpose oiled silk between the electrode and the bandage in order to prevent diffusion of the current due to the wet bandage, or else to use a rubber bandage. Some electrodes are mounted on insulated handles, made of wood or plastic, and the handle is fitted with attachments to make, break, or otherwise regulate the current. Electrodes with permanently attached or removable handles are used mainly for short applications to small areas, such as in testing for electrical responses of muscles and nerves and also for treating weak or paralyzed muscles (motor point treatment). *Cardiac catheters* contain electrodes that are threaded through veins into the chambers of the heart and are used to monitor and maintain the rhythm of the heart.

Further details on different electrodes and their handling and securing will be found in the chapters on the various currents.

MISCELLANEOUS ACCESSORIES

Treatment Timers. For the accurate measuring of treatment time, and as an added feature for safety of application, special alarm clocks or automatic clock turn-offs are well nigh indispensable. These clocks can usually be set for any number of minutes from 1 to 60. Anyone practicing physical therapy should at the very start acquire the habit of setting a clock for the treatment period for each patient. This will avoid the occasional situation when, on account of some distraction, a patient may be left too long connected to a machine or under a lamp. Most diathermy and ultrasound machines have built-in timers.

Patient's Release. A patient's release consists of a cut-off switch that can be operated by a gentle pull of a cord placed within reach of the patient. It will immediately reassure a patient who is apprehensive about an electrical treatment if he knows that he can turn off the current at any time without even calling for the doctor. As a matter of fact, with skillfully applied electrodes and proper dosage of current, there will hardly ever be any occasion to utilize such release except in a real emergency, like the slipping of a cord tip or dislodging of an electrode due to an untoward movement of the patient.

Foot Switches. For the application of treatment where both hands of the operator are needed, as in the surgical application of high-frequency currents or electrodiagnostic testing, it is important to be able to start or cut off the current by a foot switch. Foot switches are available on some generators for measuring chronaxie and strength-duration curves.

Treatment Tables and Couches. Well-built tables or couches are essential for the efficient administration of electrical and light treatments. A wooden table 26 inches high, 24 inches wide, and 72 inches long, with upholstered top and a head-rest, is the most desirable when one table has to serve for all treatment. It is suggested that either the head or the foot end be adjustable. Patients with stiff backs or extensive arthritic changes prefer a low couch, and this is also more convenient for light treatments, as it allows a greater range in adjusting the distance between the light and the patient. Metal tables, as a rule, are not desirable because of the possibility of grounding the current.

Size and Position of Electrodes. Electrodes are usually employed in pairs of equal size. If one electrode is smaller, it is called the *active* electrode, and the larger electrode is called the *dispersive* electrode. The term of indifferent or inactive electrode is incorrect, because it conveys the impression that no action takes place underneath it; the fact is that burns may readily occur under a large electrode with improper technique or by accident.

Pairs of electrodes may be applied in two ways: (1) over opposite surfaces of the body or an extremity—*transverse application;* or (2) placed on the same body plane—*longitudinal application.* Two forms of the longitudinal application are the cuff technique, when a circular or semicircular pair of electrodes is applied around an extremity, and the inductance cable or coil technique, in which an inductance coil is wound round an extremity. The latter method is used only in short-wave diathermy.

The *density of current* in a given area and its subsequent effects on the structures are determined by the size and position of electrodes and the current strength employed. A current passing from under a large electrode may have no appreciable effect, but when that same current is concentrated underneath a small electrode it may produce a very marked effect, even resulting at times in destruction of tissue.

With two electrodes of equal size, the density beneath each of them is equal; if one is twice as large as the other, the density of the current under the smaller will be twice as great as under the larger. As the current spreads between two electrodes across the body, its density must gradually decrease, so that midway between the electrodes the density is usually least. The nearer the electrodes are applied to each other, the greater will be the density of the current between them. If both electrodes are placed on the same side of the body or of a limb, the density of the current will be the greatest in the skin and in the superficial parts. The closer the electrodes are placed, the greater becomes the density between the closely adjoined edges, known as the *edge-effect.* This is first manifested by an unpleasant burning sensation and, when unheeded, may result in a superficial blister or deep burn.

When the cross section of an area between the electrodes is narrower than that of the electrodes, there is greater density of the current in the narrower path, and any undue increase of current strengths will bring forth an excess of response and pain in that area. In surgical applications, the current density under the active electrode, a needle point, is increased far beyond physiological tolerance, and tissue destruction occurs. Needle electrodes are also used, but with less intensity of current, in acupuncture.

Conductivity of Tissues.   The human body consists of a composite mass of tissues with varying electrical conductivity. The outermost layer of the skin, the stratum corneum, is composed of a horny layer, which, being a good insulator, forms the chief resistance of the body. The resistance of the skin can be considered as a measure of the resistance of the entire body. The relative conductivity of the various tissues is about equal to their content of water: muscle, 72 to 75 per cent; brain, 68 per cent; fat, 14 to 15 per cent; peripheral nerves, skin, and bone, 5 to 16 per cent. In general, tissues that contain the most water and are therefore richest in ions are the best conductors.

Muscle and brain show the best conductivity of all the tissues; muscle conducts about four times better in the longitudinal direction of its fibers than transversely. Tendons and fasciæ are poor conductors on account of their lower content of water. Peripheral nerves conduct six times as readily as muscular substances; it is difficult to utilize this advantage, however, because a nerve is usually surrounded by fat and by a fibrous sheath, and both are poor conductors. The subcutaneous tissue is a relatively good conductor. Bones are the poorest conductors, especially those of dense structure. Internal organs, such as the liver, lungs, stomach, and intestines, offer a varying degree of resistance, dependent on their relative content of blood, air, and connective tissue, and, in the case of the hollow viscera, on their contents.

The size of the electrodes and the distance between them plays an important role in skin conductivity. It is evident that the larger size of the electrodes offers larger surface for the entry of the current. This results in a decrease of skin resistance proportional to the area of application. When electricity is applied in a full water bath, large amounts can be introduced. Resistance to the current varies in direct proportion to the distance between electrodes; the longer the path the current has to travel, the more resistance it must overcome.

Electric Injuries. Accidental injuries by electricity may be caused either by electric shock, due to a sudden powerful influence of electricity on the entire body, or by electric burns, due to excessive current density over part of the body.

Electric shock may be caused by accidental contact with a grounded object such as a water pipe, radiator, or electric circuit during an electric treatment. Shock due to such contacts becomes especially serious if these occur over a large surface of the body, such as during a bath. Another more serious but extremely rare cause of electric shock is transformer breakdown, when a defect occurs in a piece of apparatus in the insulation between the primary and secondary side of the transformer and the high-tension low-frequency current jumps over to the patient. The elderly cardiac patient with conduction disturbances of the heart may have a cardiac pacemaker implanted in his chest. Great care must be taken in the application of all electrical appliances to such patients. All electrical apparatus should be checked for leakage of electricity and should be standardized periodically. The use of diathermy on such patients can be particularly dangerous.

Electric burns are brought about by an excess of electricity applied to the skin or mucous membrane. In electrosurgery, such excessive density is purposely employed to cause tissue destruction. In ordinary electrotherapy, no tissue destruction is ever desired, and the observance of the rules of safe technique will always prevent such burns. The clinical appearance of burns varies from a passing erythema to blistering of super-

5

ficial layers of the skin or deep tissue coagulation with subsequent slough-ing and ulcer formation. They are slow to heal, may become infected, and, according to the depth and the location of destruction, may be fol-lowed at times by extensive unsightly scarring.

GENERAL RULES OF TREATMENT

In order to carry out electric treatments safely and efficiently, close observation of certain basic rules is required.

1. **Method of Procedure.**   Calm and businesslike method of procedure is essential. Many patients are apprehensive when receiving electrical treatment for the first time, and a nervous, fidgety operator adds to their uneasiness. Patients should be told that electrical treatments may be uncomfortable but do not hurt and do not burn and that there is never more current administered than can be comfortably tolerated. Before patients are brought near a piece of apparatus, the operator must know that it is properly connected and in good working order and that all controls are off or in zero position.

2. **Position of Patient.**   Patients should be placed in a position in which they will remain comfortable during the entire treatment period. For treatment of the head, abdomen, pelvis and thigh, or entire lower ex-tremity, patients are best put in a recumbent position. The shoulder and upper arm should usually be treated with the arm propped up (as much abduction as possible) by pillows on a small table; the elbow and forearm should be treated resting on a table. In neck or chest treatments, patients may sit propped up in an armchair. For knee, leg, or foot treatments, an armchair with a foot-part that can be raised is convenient.

3. **Inspection of Parts.**   Before applying electrodes, carefully inspect parts to be treated to make sure that the skin looks and feels normal. Special precautions in treatment are necessary in case of recent scar tissue, in peripheral nerve injuries, and in other cases of disturbed sensa-tion. Preliminary exposure for 10 minutes to luminous heat is a good rou-tine measure to warm and relax the parts and decrease skin resistance.

4. **Placing of Electrodes and Cords.** Choose electrodes of proper type and size. Prepare low-frequency pad electrodes by moistening them with warm salt solution or water. Metal electrodes may be used with commer-cial paste, and 1-inch rubber bands hold them in place. Place electrodes in correct position, and see that they are in good contact all the way through. Secure electrodes with elastic bandages (avoid too much and too tight bandaging) or small sandbags; whenever possible, one electrode should be held by part of the body resting on it. Fasten conducting cords to the electrodes and binding posts (terminals) of the apparatus. See that electrodes and conducting cords or cable stay secure during entire treatment.

5. **Starting the Treatment.**   Everything is now ready to start the flow of current. Set the time clock or automatic switch for the prescribed treatment time. Turn on the main switch to admit the supply current. Proceed to turn on a comfortable current strength by gradually opening the controls. Warn the patient to report any unpleasant sensation—pricking, excess heat—at once. *Never leave the patient out of sight or sound once the treatment has been started,* unless the patient can instantly shut off the current if necessary.

6. **Regulation of Current Strength.**   It may take 3 to 5 minutes to reach the maximum current strength and to allow for gradual overcoming of skin resistance. The strength of current to be employed depends on the size of the active electrode, the condition to be treated, and the individual sensitivity of the patient. If the patient complains any time during treatment about pain, burning, or any other unpleasant sensation and if decreasing the current strength does not give immediate relief, turn off current entirely. After the patient is comfortable again, advance controls carefully; if the patient still complains, take off and inspect electrodes and their site, making sure that all controls are off. There may be poor contact or too much pressure under the electrodes, or the patient may simply be oversensitive. After reapplying electrodes, proceed as on first starting current; never push up current strength if the patient is not entirely comfortable. It is generally more beneficial to use a moderate amount of current for a longer period than to push up the current to the limit of toleration for a short intensive treatment.

7. **Termination of Treatment.**   Turn off controls slowly in the reverse order to that in which they were turned on. Take off electrodes only after the current has been turned off entirely. See that all controls are turned back to zero. Inspect the site of electrodes carefully. Report any unusual changes at once to the physician in charge, and make a record of them. Let patient rest for a few moments after every treatment. In inclement weather, make sure that patients are allowed 10 to 15 minutes to cool off before they go outside.

Chapter 11

THE DIRECT CURRENT AND
ION TRANSFER

Historical. The galvanic current, better described as the direct or constant current, is the basic and also the first known form of electric current flow. Galvani, professor of anatomy at the University of Bologna in Italy, noticed in 1780 that whenever a spark leapt between the electrodes of an electrical friction machine, a freshly dissected frog's leg that was lying on a metal plate suddenly twitched. But if the leg was hung on an iron grille by a copper hook, it also twitched every time it touched the grille. Galvani interpreted this as an evidence that the animal body was a source of electricity and that the metals served to discharge it. Soon thereafter, another Italian, Volta, proved that electricity arose at the contact of two different metals and caused the muscles of the leg to contract. He constructed the "voltaic pile" from alternate discs of copper and zinc, separated from each other by porous discs made of paper soaked in vinegar. This was the first electric cell ever produced. Volta's discovery was the first means of generating a constant flow of current, but the name galvanism was retained to honor the original discoverer of the phenomenon itself.

The galvanic current came into general therapeutic use at the end of the last century with the construction of wet batteries of fairly large capacity; together with the faradic current, it served for many basic observations in the physiology of nerves and muscles. Apostoli's method of treating uterine fibroids by surgical galvanism and Leduc's discovery that it is possible to introduce medicinal substances into the skin through the ionic effects of the galvanic current caused great interest for a few years, but this soon subsided, and after 1910 high-frequency currents occupied the center of the electrotherapeutic stage.

Physics and Apparatus. The galvanic or direct (also known as constant) current is an uninterrupted, unidirectional flow of electrons. It may be derived from a variety of sources.

Dry cells or *batteries* are the source of the smoothest flow of current; they also have the advantage that they are easily portable and can be used everywhere. Their essential physics have been presented in Chapter 8.

A single dry cell furnishes only a very small amount of current. A 1½-volt dry cell has an output, when working at fullest efficiency, of about 15 amperes. Usually the load is not that heavy, and the current depends upon the resistance of the circuit. It is more convenient to use the large dry batteries originally designed for radio purposes, formerly known as B batteries. They serve as an efficient source of galvanic current. In cases of emergency, several 1½-volt dry cells may be combined into a large battery. The large dry cells are available in 22½-volt and 45-volt or larger strength. Any electrician should be able to build a homemade galvanic outfit with one of these, placing it in a suitable box and connecting it in series with a rheostat and a plain milliammeter (Fig. 11–1). A rheostat is necessary to control the current strength in the circuit, and a meter allows the reading of this amount; the meter also serves to register the eventual decline of the battery. The polarity of the apparatus should be

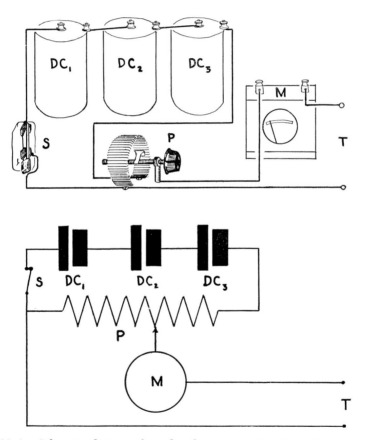

Fig. 11–1.   Schematic diagram of simple galvanic generator. Upper figure: schematic diagram of a simple galvanic circuit. Lower figure: Equivalent electrical diagram of the above figure. *DC₁, DC₂, DC₃,* dry cells in series; *P,* potentiometer; *M,* milliammeter; *T,* treatment terminals; *S,* switch.

indicated by marking the terminals plainly with + and − signs. Battery outfits are, however, available commercially at quite reasonable cost.

Vacuum or valve-tube rectifiers consist of thermionic tubes and serve to change an alternating current supply into a fairly smooth direct or galvanic current (Fig. 11–2). These rectifiers consist of a small box or cabinet containing the rectifying tube, a current regulator or rheostat, meter, terminals marked for polarity, and pole-changing switch (Fig. 11–3). They are portable and relatively inexpensive and are most frequently employed nowadays as a source of galvanism, and of the basic low-frequency currents.

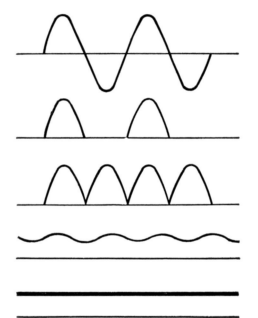

Fig. 11–2. Scheme of changing alternating into direct current by vacuum-tube or semiconductor diode rectification. The stages shown are half-wave rectification, full-wave rectification, partial filtration, and, finally, total filtration.

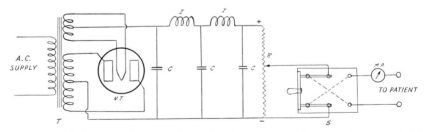

Fig. 11–3. Schematic diagram of transforming commercial alternating current into direct (galvanic) current by means of a vacuum (thermionic) tube rectifier. *T* is a transformer connected to the alternating current supply: *VT*, a vacuum tube rectifier; *C*, capacitors; *I*, choke coils; *R*, a variable resistance; *S*, reversing switch; and *MA*, milliammeter.

Semiconductor diodes or metallic rectifiers are so-called junctions of *p*-type and *n*-type semiconductors. A semiconductor is a material that will conduct electricity if any charges are present but that normally does not conduct because of an absence of free charges (intrinsic semiconductor). An *n*-type semiconductor is one that has free electrons, while *p*-type semiconductor is one that has free absences (called holes) of electrons. Under the influence of an electric field, the holes drift toward the negative pole (they act like positively charged electrons), and the electrons drift toward the positive pole. In a *p–n* junction, rectification occurs because a positive voltage applied to the *p* side of the junction will repel the holes and attract the electrons. A negative voltage applied to the *p* side of the junction will attract the holes and repel the electrons, and the space between the *p* and *n* regions will become completely depleted of charge and will act like an insulator. This easier passage of electrons in one direction than in the other serves as an additional means of changing alternating current into direct current.

Motor generators consist of a combination of a motor and a dynamo. The motor is either an alternating or direct current motor, and it rotates the dynamo, which furnishes the galvanic current and also usually a number of low-frequency currents. For the production of a smooth direct current, additional capacitors and choke coils are incorporated.

Polarity. The galvanic current is the only current applied according to "polarity." All generators of a galvanic current have two terminals or poles, a positive and a negative one. In all forms of galvanic treatments in which an "active" or therapeutically effective electrode is employed, it must be connected to the pole required by the condition treated. Hence the operator must at times be sure which is the positive and which is the negative pole or terminal. Dry cells, rectifier tubes, and motor generators are of "fixed" polarity, that is, the terminals of the apparatus are marked positive (+) or negative (−); if it is desirable to change their polarity, a suitable switch arrangement always clearly indicates the positive and negative poles.

Testing for Polarity. Fasten two conducting cords to the two terminals of a galvanic source and drop the distal tips about 2 inches apart in a flat vessel containing tap water to which a pinch of salt has been added. As soon as a little current is turned on, white bubbles appear rapidly and in great numbers around one cord tip. The pole that causes the rapid bubbling is the negative pole (cathode); the bubbles consist of hydrogen gas. After a while, a few large bubbles appear slowly at the other cord tip, the positive pole (anode); these bubbles consist of oxygen. This polarity action of the direct current is invariably characteristic for each of its poles; if by a "pole-changer" the direction of current flow is reversed and the experiment is repeated, the rapid bubble formation will take place at the opposite cord tip. Thus the negative pole can always be

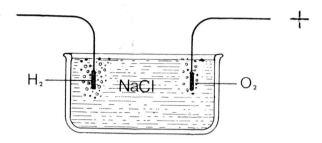

Fig. 11–4. Testing for polarity of galvanic generator.

readily determined by the quick appearance of many small bubbles (Fig. 11–4).

Another simple test for polarity is the phenolphthalein test: A piece of blotting paper is moistened with a dilute phenolphthalein solution. When it is touched with the two cord tips with a slight amount of current flowing, a red dot appears at the negative pole.

Physicochemical and Physiological Effects (Table 11–1). Although the direct current is the simplest current so far as physics is concerned, the explanation of its mode of action upon the body is somewhat complicated.

The human body may be considered from the viewpoint of electrotherapy as a bag of skin holding a solution of common salt (NaCl). When the molecules of NaCl dissolve in water, they dissociate into sodium ions (Na^+) bearing a positive charge and chlorine ions (Cl^-) bearing a negative charge. The flow of a direct current through the salt solution causes these ions to move in a definite direction, the sodium ions migrating toward the negative pole (cathode) and the chlorine ions toward the positive pole (anode); this process is known as *ion transfer* (iontophoresis). When the positively charged sodium ions arrive at the negative pole and the negatively charged chlorine ions arrive at the positive pole, they lose their charge and become free unelectrified atoms; these in turn cause a secondary chemical reaction: the formation of caustic sodium hydroxide and liberation of hydrogen at the negative pole, and formation of caustic hydrochloric acid and liberation of oxygen at the positive pole. The principal physical effect of ion transfer by the direct current is an acid reaction at the positive and an alkaline one at the negative pole; the intensity of each reaction varies with the strength and relative density of the current at each pole. This acid and alkaline effect may be described as a polar effect because it occurs only under the electrodes.

In addition to the polar effect caused by ion transfer, nondissociated colloid molecules, such as droplets of fat, albumin, particles of starch, blood cells, bacteria, and other single cells, all of which have an electrical charge due to the adsorption of ions, also move under the influence of a direct current toward the negative pole; this is known as *cataphoresis*.

Table 11–1. Effects of the Direct Current

	Physicochemical	Physiological
Positive pole (anode)	Acid reaction; repels metals and alkaloids	Hardening of tissues; decrease of nerve irritability
Negative pole (cathode)	Alkaline reaction; repels acids and acid radicals	Softening of tissues; increase of nerve irritability
Both poles	Mild heating	Vasomotor stimulation

Finally, there also occurs a shifting of the water content of the tissues through membrane structures with an electrical charge known as *electro-osmosis*. All this makes it evident that the passage of the direct current across or around cell membranes of variable permeability and along fluids of different conductivity and ionic composition presents a complicated biophysical process. There is also a minimal thermal effect.

The following demonstration serves to illustrate the physiological effect of a direct current: Place two moist-pad electrodes, well soaked in saline solution, upon opposite sides of the knee joint, start a flow of current from a galvanic source, according to the general technique described, and keep it up at comfortable toleration for 20 minutes. (With electrodes 3 by 3 inches in correct equidistant position, the average patient should tolerate from 6 to 9 milliamperes of current.) When the current starts, there will be gentle tingling and pricking under the electrodes; as the resistance of the skin decreases gradually, more current can be tolerated and the pricking sensation changes to a feeling of gentle warmth. When the electrodes are taken off at the end of the treatment, the skin will show a marked redness that is sharply restricted to the area covered by the electrodes. This color will last from 10 minutes to ½ hour.

The "galvanic hyperemia" just described is due to a chemical stimulation of the capillaries of the skin (vasomotor effect). If, hours later, another stimulus, such as a hot bath, is applied to the parts previously treated, the intensive hyperemia may reappear. It is reasonable to expect that with vasomotor stimulation lasting several hours, repeated galvanic treatment may keep up the stimulative effect and promote better blood flow not only in the skin, but possibly also in the deeper tissues.

It is important to understand that as long as electrodes of equal size are applied, the vasomotor effect by a galvanic current is the same under each electrode; furthermore, as long as there is enough moist padding kept between the metal of the electrode and the skin and the current is kept within comfortable toleration, no caustic effects will occur. On the other hand, if, instead of electrodes of equal size, one "active" electrode of the size of a small disc or needle point is applied, while the other electrode is a larger "dispersing" one, there will be a definite acid or alkaline reaction confined to the area of the active electrode: a characteristic softening effect if the active electrode is negative or a drying or hardening effect if the active electrode is positive. If the current is sufficiently strong, the effect may be a real alkaline or acid cauterization of the part, accompanied by an intense feeling of burning under the active electrode.

Another physiological effect of the galvanic current is increased nerve irritability under the negative pole and decreased irritability under the positive one, as shown by classic laboratory experiments on fresh muscle-nerve preparations. From these experiments, earlier clinicians pronounced the dogma that the negative pole of the galvanic current is stimulative and the positive pole is sedative in painful conditions. Newer investigations have shown, however, that in the human body where a nerve is situated deep in tissues of much less electrical resistance, not enough current passes to affect the nerve directly. Hence it makes no difference, so far as deeply situated nerves are concerned, whether they are treated from the positive or negative pole. In routine electrodiagnostic examinations of accessible nerves and muscles, the negative pole should be used as the stimulating pole.

The most important physicochemical effect of a direct current is the fact that when it passes through a chemical solution, it causes a migration of its component ions in a definite direction; those with a positive charge are attracted to the negative pole and those with a negative charge are attracted to the positive pole. As a large number of drugs are soluble in water, and thus are in an ionic state, one can introduce the ions of such drugs into the skin or mucous membranes by the polarity effect of a direct current. All that is needed is to saturate a pad electrode with the solution, connect it to the proper pole and start the current flowing. This is known as ionic medication, iontophoresis, or medicinal ion transfer. Leduc's classic experiments on ion transfer are shown in Figures 11–5 and 11–6.

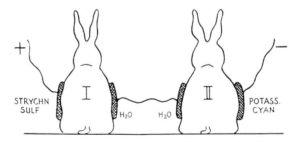

Fig. 11–5. Leduc's classic experiment. Two rabbits are placed in series in the same direct current, so that the current has to pass through both. The current enters the first rabbit by a positive electrode soaked in strychnine sulfate and leaves by a negative electrode soaked with plain water; it enters the second rabbit by an anode soaked with water and leaves by a cathode of potassium cyanide. When a current of 40 or 50 milliamperes is turned on, the first rabbit is seized by tetanic convulsions due to introduction of the strychnine ion, while the second rabbit dies rapidly with symptoms of cyanide poisoning. If the two animals are replaced by new ones and the flow is reversed, the animals are not harmed, because now the strychnine ion is not repelled by the positive pole and the cyanide not repelled by the negative pole.

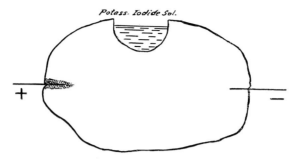

Fig. 11–6.   Potato experiment. While direct current flows, it attracts the iodine anion toward the positive pole and the free iodine there forms blue starch iodine.

Clinical Uses.   A direct current is employed for treatment purposes in three main forms: (1) medical galvanism, the use of the galvanic or direct current without introducing drugs; (2) iontophoresis, or medicinal ion transfer, the use of the direct current for the introduction of drugs or medicinal ions; (3) surgical galvanism or electrolysis, the use of the caustic polar effects of the direct current for the destruction of tissue, principally for the removal of superfluous hair.

THE DIRECT CURRENT

Therapeutic Use.   The direct current causes vasomotor stimulation of the skin and increased local circulation of the parts between the electrodes. The generally accepted explanation of the therapeutic effect is that an increase in circulation hastens the resolution of acute and chronic inflammatory products. On this basis the direct current has been used in a number of the more chronic and stubborn inflammatory conditions such as selected cases of arthritis, neuritis, and neuralgia. It is no longer a popular method of treatment in spite of the favored use of electricity as a psychotherapeutic agent. However, it continues in use as a diagnostic aid.

Technique.   The direct current is applied with moist-pad electrodes corresponding in size with that of the region to be treated. Electrodes of equal size are preferable; with such electrodes, no special attention has to be paid to polarity, and it makes no difference to which pole each electrode is connected. The interposition of a moist pad between the plate and skin is necessary for overcoming skin resistance, for protection of the skin by absorbing the caustic metallic compounds formed on the surface of the metal plate, and for maintaining perfect contact. The smooth flow of current depends on the thorough moistening and good apposition of the pads and on their safe retention. Moistening of electrodes is best done by holding them first under running warm water; after they are thoroughly soaked, they should be placed in a flat vessel containing a warm saline solution. This brings the pads to the required temperature, and after gently squeezing out the excess water, they are placed over the parts to be treated. They are held by an elastic bandage, preferably a rubber one.

Patients sensitive to cold and to moisture will complain if the electrodes are not applied at a comfortable temperature or are too wet, causing oozing over the body and clothing. It is helpful to cover the pads with a bath towel during treatment. Insufficient moistening of the pads will cause them to dry out during treatment and may give rise to imperfect conduction. If the patient complains of unpleasant burning at any time during treatment, and the amount of current does not seem excessive, the first thought is insufficient moistening of the pads causing undue current density in one spot. The remedy is to shut off the current, take off the pads, remoisten them, and reapply them carefully.

The current strength must be always within comfortable toleration of the patient. As an average, the normal skin tolerates about ½ to 1 milliampere of galvanic current per square inch of electrode surface. The size of electrodes furnishes, therefore, a guide to the expected current toleration. The smaller the electrodes, the greater the current density, and the less current can be applied. As the treatment is continued, skin resistance and the sensitivity of superficial nerve endings lessen and toleration of the current increases. It can often be observed that the meter needle advances by itself. With electrodes of suitable size, up to 30 milliamperes of current may be employed.

The duration of treatment should be from 15 to 20 minutes. Patients should never be allowed to get off the table and go out on the street with the underwear or clothing wet from treatment electrodes.

The galvanic current can be also applied to the entire surface of the body in the form of a galvanic bath.

ION TRANSFER OR IONTOPHORESIS

Therapeutic Uses. The caustic ions of the heavy metals zinc and copper may be employed in the treatment of some skin infections and chronic infections of sinuses and cavities. Chlorine ions may be employed for the loosening of superficial scars. Vasodilating drugs are chiefly used in rheumatic affections. Skin anesthesia can be produced by iontophoresis of local anesthetic drugs using the positive pole. Many drugs used for general metabolic or specific hormonal effects can be driven into the circulating blood by iontophoresis; however, most physicians employ simpler methods of using drugs.

It must be remembered that, as a rule, medicinal ions cannot be made to migrate far below the surface of the skin and mucous membranes, for they are usually precipitated.

General Technique. Any source of direct current will suffice. The correct polarity of the two terminals of the generator must be known and electrodes connected to the proper terminals. For treatment through the skin, an active pad electrode is made of sufficient thickness of absorptive material to hold the solution and to keep moist during the treatment. Gauze of a thickness of $\frac{1}{2}$ inch (about 16 layers) is best, but cotton or asbestos paper may also serve. For the introduction of vasodilating drugs, blotting paper or gauze is employed. The active electrode is soaked in the comfortably warm solution. The strength of all solutions should be 1 per cent or less; no advantage is gained by making it stronger. The saturated pad is laid on with firm contact over the area to be treated. A metal plate of somewhat smaller size is placed upon this pad very carefully, so that the metal edge nowhere touches the skin; even a minute direct contact between the metal and the skin may lead to a chemical burn.

For a dispersive electrode, a pad electrode of larger size than the active electrode is soaked in hot water or saline solution and is placed in firm contact with a convenient part of the body surface. A foot or arm bath may also be used as a dispersive electrode in all forms of treatment.

It is important that if treatment pads are to be used again, they be thoroughly cleansed and rinsed after each treatment in order to get rid of the secondary chemical products near the metal plate.

Ions with a positive charge—zinc, copper, and alkaloids such as the vasodilating drugs—are introduced into the skin and mucous membranes from the positive pole, while ions with a negative charge, like iodine, chlorine, and salicylic acid, are introduced into the tissues from the negative pole.

Copper ion transfer is applied in the treatment of chronic fungus infections of feet or hands through an "active" electrode connected to the positive pole in a copper sulfate bath, while a suitably sized dispersive pad is applied to the abdomen or the back and connected to the negative pole.

Zinc ion transfer utilizing a solution of either zinc sulfate or zinc chloride may be employed in treatment of indolent ulcers.

The treatment with copper and zinc iontophoresis is from 10 to 15 minutes at a current strength of 5 to 15 milliamperes, according to the size of the active electrode.

Histamine is a vasodilator substance that is ordinarily formed in the skin as a result of thermal, chemical, or mechanical irritation. When introduced in solution by the positive pole of a direct current, a few minutes' application will result in intense hyperemia, formation of wheals and large patches of urticaria, accompanied by a rise of 3° to 5° F in the skin temperature. This reaction subsides after a while. The resulting counterirritation has been found beneficial in the treatment of traumatic and rheumatic affections of soft tissues, such as fibrositis and neuritis.

The most frequently used technique of histamine ion transfer is to rub in a small amount of a 1 per cent histamine ointment in the skin and cover it with a moist-pad electrode connected to the positive pole, while a dispersive pad is connected to the negative pole; the current is passed for 3 to 5 minutes at 5 to 10 milliamperes strength.

Mecholyl is a derivative of choline, a vasodilating substance that stimulates the parasympathetic nerves and is an antagonist to atropine. When introduced by ion transfer from the positive pole, mecholyl causes immediate prickling of the skin followed by intense local hyperemia and perspiration of the treated area, lasting for 6 to 8 hours. After 10 minutes' treatment, mecholyl may penetrate the skin and cause general effects.

These methods are now *obsolete,* the preference being for proper surgical methods and antibiotics systemically if indicated.

Dangers.   The chief danger in all such treatments is the occurrence of skin burns or excessive destruction of the mucous membrane; these are always due to excessive density of current. It is inadvisable to depend on pain sensation as a criterion for prevention of burns; rather, current strength must always be evaluated in relation to the size of the electrodes. Another potent cause of burns is the touching of the skin by the electrode metal, insufficient padding, or denuded areas in the skin. If the metal touches the skin, burns are produced by a much lower current, evidently because of excessive current density at the point of contact.

In mecholyl iontophoresis, excessive dosage or individual sensitivity may cause unwanted systemic reaction.

Safety Rules.   In addition to the general rules of treatment described, the observation of the following *special* rules will safeguard the patient in all direct current and electrophoretic treatments.

1. Be sure that the patient's skin sensation is normal; if it is not, calculate and control the current strength carefully in accordance with the size of electrodes and the milliammeter reading.

2. Do not apply the current over denuded areas, and be most careful over recent scar tissue.

3. See that the metal plate of the electrode is evenly covered by the padding and that there are no bare edges in contact with the skin.

4. See that the covering pad is evenly soaked with tap water or saline solution.

5. Apply electrodes in good contact and with even pressure. Uneven pressure from tight bandaging or from folds or creases in the pad and insufficiently moistened areas lead to uneven distribution of current, the first subjective manifestation of which is a burning sensation in one or more spots. If the patient complains of burning at any time during treatment and the amount of current does not seem excessive, the first thought is uneven current distribution or insufficient moistening of the pads. The remedy is to shut off the current, take off the pads, remoisten them, and reapply them carefully.

6. Fasten the conducting cords securely to the electrodes, making sure that the metal of the cord tip does not come in contact with the bare skin at any point.

7. Always advance current gently when starting; never close the current sharply while the milliammeter registers current flow.

8. Be sure that the patient understands that he is to report undue burning or pain at once. The individual judgment of patients as to what they feel as burning or pain varies considerably, so that it is a safe rule never to apply more current than the patient states is comfortable, no matter what the milliampere reading shows; but, on the other hand, never exceed the safe milliammeter reading, in relation to electrode size, even if the patient claims that he can stand more current. One should bear in mind that in the course of galvanic treatments, the meter reading has a tendency to mount as skin resistance decreases. If the opposite occurs, it is usually a sign that the pads are becoming dry and need remoistening.

9. If at any time the patient complains of annoying symptoms, decrease the strength of current; if this does not afford relief, turn off the current entirely, take off the electrodes, and investigate.

10. After conclusion of treatment, do not allow patient to go outdoors with underwear or other clothing wet from the treatment.

ADDITIONAL READING

Harris, R.: Iontophoresis, pp. 146–168. In S. Licht (ed.), *Therapeutic Electricity and Ultraviolet Radiation.* 2nd ed. Licht, New Haven, Conn., 1967.

S. Licht (ed.): *Therapeutic Electricity and Ultraviolet Radiation.* 2nd ed. Licht, New Haven, Conn., 1967.

Stillwell, G. K.: Electrical stimulation and iontophoresis. In F. H. Krusen, F. J. Kottke, and P. M. Ellwood, Jr. (ed.). *Handbook of Physical Medicine and Rehabilitation.* W. B. Saunders Co., Philadelphia, 1965.

PART V

Low-Frequency Currents

Chapter 12

ELECTROPHYSIOLOGY

Bioelectric Phenomena. Electrical potentials are associated with all living tissues. The development of our present-day concepts of nerve activity has depended on improvement in electrical and electronic techniques. Each development in recording technique has made its contributions to electrophysiology, and this is especially true of vacuum tube or transistor amplification. Recording instruments have evolved from the Einthoven string galvanometer to the cathode ray oscilloscope. This newer knowledge not only allows a better understanding of the principles of electrodiagnosis, but also enables some interpretation of the possible effects of electromedical currents on the structures of the body, especially in low-frequency stimulation of muscles. Hence it seems appropriate that, as an introduction to the physiological basis of electrodiagnosis, some of the bioelectric phenomena connected with vital processes be discussed.

ACTION POTENTIALS

Membrane Potentials. An electrical potential exists across the membranes of almost all resting cells of the body. This potential has its origin in the movement and unequal distribution of ions across the cell membrane of the nerve or muscle fiber. An excess number of negative ions accumulates immediately inside the cell membrane along its inner surface, and an equal number of positive ions accumulates along the outside surface of the membrane. A state of negativity on the inside and of positivity on the outside creates a difference of potential known as the membrane potential. The mechanism for the development of a membrane potential depends upon the diffusion of some ions and the active transport of other ions across the cell membrane.

The momentary difference in electric potential between active and resting parts of a nerve fiber or muscle is known as the *action potential*. It can be demonstrated by connecting the two parts with a sensitive galvanometer. To record these potentials, it is necessary to employ nonpolarized electrodes, in which the metallic electrode is dipped into a solution containing its own ions, e.g., chloridized silver wires dipped in a chloride solution. This solution is separated from the sodium chloride

139

solution of the tissues by a porous material such as kaolin. Such an arrangement prevents a "polarization" current from the liberated hydrogen and dissolved metal in ordinary electrodes, which complicates the depolarization phenomena associated with excitation.

Action Potentials of Skeletal Muscles. In the human body, it is possible to record the action potentials resulting from voluntary muscular contraction. If coaxial needle electrodes are inserted into the muscle, the activity of a single motor unit is recorded. Surface electrodes are used to record from the whole muscle. The single action potential is a wave of short duration in the range of one millisecond with the characteristics of a spike. In a muscle at rest under conditions of complete relaxation, there are no currents recorded with standard techniques. During gentle muscular contractions, the motor units discharge in a range between 6 and 60 per cent, the amplitude and frequency increasing with the strength of contraction (Fig. 12–1). The individual motor units discharge independently and asynchronously. The entire muscle discharges at a higher frequency, about 300 per second, during a muscle tetanus.

Action Potentials in Nerves. With the use of the electromyograph, action potentials of nerves have been studied (Fig. 12–2), and their conduction along individual nerve fibers, rather than whole nerves, has been investigated, and it has been found that different types of nerve fibers have different rates of conduction. Physiologists have long known that the excitement of a nerve is followed by certain definite periods of excitability. On stimulation, a physicochemical change takes place in the nerve for a very

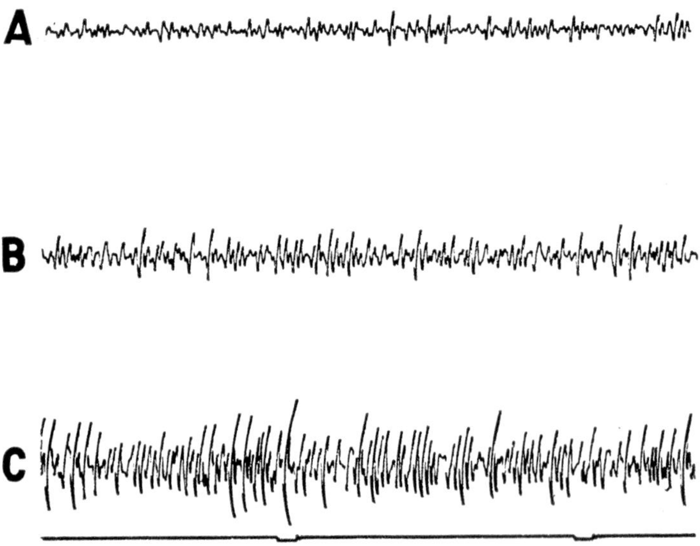

Fig. 12–1. Normal muscle with skin electrodes. Electromyogram of gentle (A), moderate (B), and strong (C) contraction. Time interval 1 second on bottom signal.

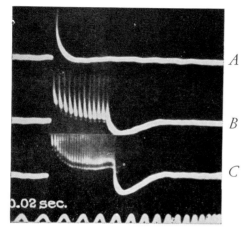

A

B

C

0.02 sec.

Fig. 12–2. Cathode-ray-recorded action potentials in a phrenic nerve. *A*, single shock; *B*, brief tetanus at 180 per second; *C*, brief tetanus at 350 per second. Temperature 37° C. Note development of positive afterpotential. (Gasser, H. S.: The Control of Excitation in the Nervous System. Harvey Lectures. Williams & Wilkins Company, 1937, p. 176.)

short interval of time, during which no further excitement is possible. This period is known as the *absolute refractory period* and lasts about 1 msec. Following this is a variable period of up to 15 msec during which the nerve recovers its conductivity, first rather rapidly and then more gradually. This is the *relative refractory period*. This period is often followed by the supernormal period during which the nerve is most excitable. The highest frequency of stimulation to which a nerve is able to respond depends upon the length of its refractory period. Thus, an absolute refractory period of 1 msec limits the rate stimulation to 1,000 impulses per second. Some of the larger myelinated axons respond to a current of 2,000 impulses per second and hence must have an absolute refractory period of about 0.5 msec. The maximum frequencies noted in motor nerves carrying natural impulses is about 400 per second. This gives a rather large factor of tolerance for the rate of the stimulating current.

All somatic nerves are large bundles of mixed fibers of varying kinds. The sciatic nerve of a frog, for example, contains about 4,000 myelinated and about 8,000 unmyelinated fibers. Each type of fiber has a specific conduction rate. Cathode-ray studies have shown three types of waves, A, B, and C. A-waves travel along a nerve bundle at the rate of 30 to 90 meters per second, B-waves at the rate of 15 to 25 meters per second, and C-waves at the rate of 1 to 2 meters per second. Motor fibers are known to have predominantly the A type of conduction. Sensory fibers at the dorsal root show a mixture of all three types of conduction, while the sympathetic gray rami show types B and C.

Action Potentials of the Heart and the Brain. It has been known since 1856 that the contraction of the heart was associated with a change of electric potential, and in 1903 Einthoven invented the delicate string electrocardiograph with a camera to photograph its deflections. *Electrocardiography* has since that time assumed a major role in the diagnosis of heart conditions.

In recent years, it was recognized that all functional activities of the cortex of the brain are associated with electric changes, and *electroencephalography* plays an increasingly important role in the understanding of the function of the brain and in the diagnosis of the disorders of the central nervous system.

Theory of Bioelectric Phenomena. The electrical potential differences following excitation may be explained either by movement of ions across polarized membranes or by a sudden fall of potential across the membrane.

In theory, the nerve (or muscle) fiber membrane is provided with a sodium pump and a potassium pump, which maintain a differential concentration of sodium and potassium ions, respectively, inside and outside the nerve fiber. Also, the permeability of the membrane is selective to sodium and potassium ions but impermeable to the diffusion of large numbers of organic and protein ions inside the nerve fiber. Thus the resting membrane potential is brought about, and the membrane is said to be polarized. Any factor that increases the permeability of the membrane to sodium ions is likely to elicit a sequence of rapid changes in membrane potential lasting only thousandths of a second, after which an immediate return of the membrane potential to its resting value ensues. This sequence of potential changes is called the *action potential.* Some of the factors that can elicit an action potential are electrical stimulation, heat, cold; or anything that momentarily disturbs the normal resting state of the membrane (Guyton, 1972).

Depolarization and Repolarization. The action potential occurs in two separate stages—depolarization and repolarization. Ions move across the polarized membrane when the permeability of the membrane is disturbed by a mechanical, electrical, or chemical stimulus. Sodium ions rush to the inside of the fiber, carrying enough positive charges inside to cause complete disappearance of the normal resting potential. There is now a reversal of potential, with a negative state outside and a positive state inside. Immediately after depolarization takes place, the membrane becomes almost totally impermeable to sodium ions and the normal resting membrane potential returns. This is called repolarization.

ELECTRICAL STIMULATION OF NERVES AND MUSCLES

Nature of Nerve Impulses. A stimulus or excitant biologically represents a change in environment, either naturally or artificially introduced. In the body, these generally consist of chemical or physical influences that produce polarity changes at membrane interfaces with sufficient rapidity to stimulate a cell to action. Electrical stimuli, when properly used and controlled, most nearly approximate natural physiological impulses. The effectiveness of an electrical stimulus depends on its intensity, its form and the duration of its effective period.

When a nerve is excited naturally or artificially by a stimulus, i.e., by a sudden change in its environment, a local disturbance is set up that is propagated in both directions from the point of stimulation. This is variously designated as the nerve impulse, the excitation wave, or the propagated disturbance. It differs fundamentally from physical waves and mechanical oscillations in two ways: (*a*) The energy for progression is derived not from the energy of the stimulus but from successive physical and chemical changes in the fiber over which it travels; and (*b*) it is conducted without loss of intensity, i.e., without decrement. The velocity of impulse conduction in motor nerves in general has been found to be 40 to 100 meters per second in mammals.

The independent irritability of muscles was first demonstrated by the classic experiment of Claude Bernard, who injected an infusion of curare into the dorsal lymph sac of a frog. The animal became paralyzed and the stimulation of motor nerves by single electrical impulses caused no contraction, while direct stimulation of the muscle evoked a normal response. The prevalent opinion is that in normal muscles an electrical current stimulates muscle cells directly, as well as exciting twigs of nerve fibers in the muscular mass.

All forms of voluntary *muscular contraction are tetanic.* Stimuli originate in the pyramidal cells of the cerebral cortex, are propagated by a

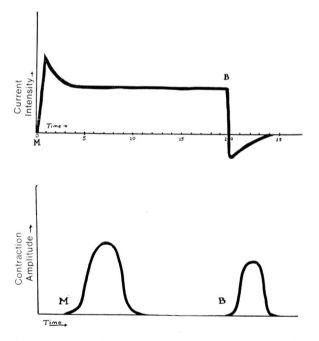

Fig. 12–3.   Response of normal muscle to stimulation by direct or galvanic current. *M*, make; *B*, break. Response occurs only at peaks between 0 and 3 and 20 and 23 and is weaker on break than on make.

long axon down the spinal cord, and pass over synaptic junctions with the dendrites of spinal cord cells. In this way, the excitation process, initiated in the central neuron, excites the cell bodies of the peripheral neurons. From the spinal motor neurons, impulses are transmitted to the muscle fibers by axons leaving the spinal cord. It is well known that such voluntary contractions are not twitches or jerks; on the contrary, they are smooth, graded, sustained, and larger contractions that result in graceful movements of the bony levers to which they are attached. Such contractions are due to the fact that the pyramidal cells send out not a single stimulus but successive volleys of impulses that are graded in frequency and duration. They are said to enter the muscle at a rate of 5 to 100 per second.

Stimulation by Direct Current. If a galvanic (direct) current is suddenly started or interrupted ("made" or "broken") over muscular parts or motor nerves, there occurs a muscular contraction or phenomenon of a sensory character (slight shock), at first under the electrode connected to the negative pole and, with a suitable increase of current strength, also under the electrode connected to the positive pole (Fig. 12–3).

The law of electrical muscle and nerve stimulation as first formulated by DuBois-Reymond states that the intensity of a stimulus and the subsequent muscular contraction are directly proportional to the magnitude and change in current strength (voltage and amperage) or, in the presence of same current strength, the intensity is proportional to the rate of fluctuation (the rapidity with which it occurs). Nernst first promulgated the theory that stimulation of muscles and nerves was due to changes in ionic concentration at the cell membrane. Changes in the membrane potential occur in accordance with the strength of the current and its duration. Differences in concentration act as stimuli until they are equalized by a process of diffusion. The steadily flowing galvanic current causes no muscular contraction because there is not enough change in its strength or its rate of fluctuation to act as a stimulus.

Electrotonus. The closing ("make") of a direct current on a nerve produces an increase of irritability at the negative pole or cathode (*cathelectrotonus*) and a decrease of irritability at the positive pole or anode (*analectrotonus*). This is Pfluger's well-known law and can now be explained by our knowledge of bioelectric currents. The closing contractions, elicited with weak and moderate stimuli, are due to a depolarization at the anode.

It is important to know that the changes of irritability that develop immediately on closing a current do not persist in a static state while the current continues to flow. Furthermore, if the anode and cathode are applied over human nerves, the effects are complicated by the spread of current through the tissues, as shown in Figure 12–4. As is easily visualized, under each physical anode and cathode (A–C) there exist what may be termed a pair of physiological anodes and cathodes (*ac* and *a'c'*).

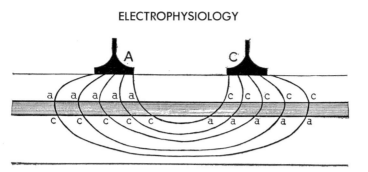

Fig. 12–4.   Diagram illustrating effects of the anode and cathode on human nerves. A, C, physical poles of electrodes applied to skin; a, c, physiological poles in underlying nerve—a and c beneath C correspond to a′ and c′ in text description.

When the current is closed, the excitation could develop at either physiological cathode (c or c′), but as the density of the current is greater at c′, the closing contraction originates at this point. As the current strength is increased, it also develops at c. Stronger currents are required, however, to produce excitation at the physiological anodes a and a′, but as the density of current is greater at a than at a′, it will arise at a′ last and only when currents are exceedingly strong.

We may therefore align the sequence of responses as follows, with regard to the physiological poles: c′ and c on closing, a and a′ on opening. In practice, however, the physical electrodes (A and C) are employed; hence the sequence:

> Cathode closing contraction (CCC),
> Anode closing contraction (ACC),
> Anode opening contraction (AOC),
> Cathode opening contraction (COC).

Although the responses may vary greatly with the current intensity, it is customary to use the cathode in routine stimulation since it takes less current and is therefore more comfortable.

Nerve Block.   Passage of an impulse through a nerve can be impeded or prevented entirely by mechanical or chemical agents as well as by the anodal effects of the direct current. This means that functional block can be produced without cutting or injuring the fibers permanently. The "electrotonic" interruption of the conduction of stimulation occurs only with stronger currents and is considered to be due to the effects of deep secondary chemical and colloidal processes on the nerve membrane that cause a reversal of the normal process of irritability.

Electrical Excitability.   The power of a muscle to respond to an electrical stimulus is a complex function dependent on a number of variable factors that make quantitative measurements difficult. The muscle contraction will vary according to the intensity of the electric current applied, the duration of the stimulus, and the rate of development of the current.

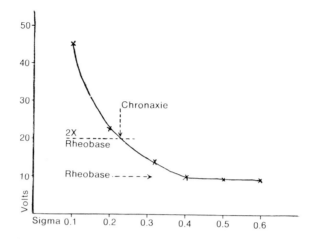

Fig. 12–5. Diagram illustrating excitation time, rheobase, and chronaxie.

Irritability is also altered by changes in the length of a muscle or the degree of stretch. Insofar as possible, these variables must be controlled or measured when testing muscle excitability.

Strength-Duration Curves. In clinical practice, a minimal or threshold contraction is chosen as the index of response, as it can be more accurately repeated than a submaximal response, and maximal stimuli are usually too painful to be tolerated. The rate of propagation of the stimulating current or its wave form may be held constant, depending on the choice of stimulator. The two variables remaining are the intensity of the stimulus and its duration. The excitability of muscle can be determined, then, by taking a constant index of response and a constant wave form of stimulating current and measuring the intensity of current required to produce the response when it is applied for a measured duration. The results of such measurements at varying intensity and duration of stimulus may be plotted in the form of a strength-duration curve that gives a graphic index of excitability (Fig. 12–5).

Several different types of stimulators may be used for this purpose, including rheotomes, condenser discharges, or, more recently, electronic stimulators that produce currents of rectilinear wave form.

Chronaxie. If a long duration or constant current is used to stimulate a muscle or nerve, the intensity that is just sufficient to cause a threshold contraction has been called by Lapicque the *rheobase*. He also introduced the idea of doubling the rheobasic current arbitrarily and of determining the shortest time interval that it must act in order to produce a minimal contraction. This time is called *chronaxie*. By referring to the graph of the strength-duration curve, it can be seen that the chronaxie of a tissue is determined by measuring an arbitrary point on the curve. It is obvious that chronaxie is a reciprocal of excitability; decreased chronaxie signifies increased excitability and *vice versa*. Chronaxie determination has become of practical importance in electrodiagnosis as a fairly exact index of excitability, although it does not give as complete information as the whole strength-duration curve.

Progressive Currents. As previously mentioned, the response of a muscle to stimulation by an electric current is influenced by the rate of propagation of the current as well as by the intensity and duration. Experimental work has shown that in normal muscles, as the current gradient decreases, the current strength required for excitation increases. Currents that increase linearly or exponentially are called progressive currents and have been used both for electrodiagnosis and for treatment of denervated muscle.

Intensity-Frequency Relation. Another measure of excitability has been the response of nerve and muscle to sinusoidal alternating currents of different frequencies. With this type of current, both the duration of the stimulus and the rate of rise vary according to the frequency. At high frequencies, the gradient is steep and the duration brief, while at low frequencies, the rise is slow and the duration long.

Tetanus-Frequency Relation. A similar measurement may be made by stimulating with rectangular wave impulses of 50-msec duration and varying the frequency. That frequency which produces a tetanic muscular contraction is recorded. This relation is helpful in differentiating normal from denervated muscle.

Galvanic Tetanus Ratio. Normal muscle, when stimulated briefly with a direct current, responds with a brisk twitch. If the intensity is increased to 10 or 12 times the rheobase value, a sustained contraction or mild tetanus results.

Denervated muscle has a slow contraction on direct current stimulation that resembles a tetanic contraction. The ratio between the intensity of a direct current sufficient to cause tetanus and that causing a twitch is the galvanic tetanus ratio. In the normal muscle, it may be 10 or 12 to 1, but in the denervated muscle, the ratio is near 1 to 1.

ADDITIONAL READING

Goodgold, J., and Eberstein, A.: *Electrodiagnosis of Neuromuscular Diseases.* The Williams & Wilkins Co., Baltimore, 1972.

Guyton, A. C.: *Organ Physiology, Structure and Function of the Nervous System* W. B. Saunders Co., Philadelphia, 1972.

Katz, B.: *Nerve, Muscle, and Synapse.* McGraw-Hill Book Co., New York, 1966.

Chapter 13

ELECTRODIAGNOSIS

General Considerations. Electrodiagnosis deals with the reaction of muscles and motor nerves to electrical stimuli. It furnishes a valuable aid from the standpoint of diagnosis, prognosis, and therapy in pathological conditions of the motor tract, including the brain, the spinal cord, and the peripheral nerves and also the muscles.

Electrical stimulation of muscles and nerves has for over a century formed part of the large field of physiology. The principle of electrodiagnosis was discovered by a Frenchman, Duchenne, and was further developed by French and German physiologists, among them Erb, Remak, Pflüger, DuBois-Reymond, and Babinski, until the classical method of testing by the faradic and galvanic currents was fully established. Later investigators, including Lapicque, Bourguignon, and Adrian, developed more modern methods of greater precision.

Electromyography was developed by Piper, Bronk, and Matthews and consists of the recording and measurement of the voltages generated by normal and abnormal muscles. The most recent method for study of electrical activity is conduction velocity in peripheral nerves, first introduced by Hodes *et al.* in 1948. Electromyography appears to be the method of choice as a diagnostic aid.

We have seen in the foregoing electrophysiological considerations that each skeletal muscle possesses the property of independent irritability and contractility if artificial stimuli are directly applied to it. Likewise, any nerve fiber may be stimulated by artificial means at any point in its course. Electrical stimulation is the most effective and convenient artificial stimulant of both muscle and nerve. A suitable electrical stimulus applied to a motor nerve elicits a contraction in all of the muscles supplied by the nerve distal to the point of stimulation. A suitable electrical stimulus applied to a muscle elicits a contraction of the muscle itself and may also spread to the neighboring muscles. The character of the response varies with the nature and strength of the stimulus employed and the normal or pathological state of the nerve or muscle.

Many of the pathological conditions in the central and peripheral nervous system are accompanied by typical changes in the electrical reaction (Table 13–1). It may be normal, it may be exaggerated, it may be

Table 13-1. Changes in Electrical Reactions

Quantitative changes	(a) Hyperexcitability
	(b) Hypoexcitability
Qualitative	(a) Contraction sluggish
	(b) Contraction persists
	(c) Contraction quickly ceases
Qualitative-quantitative	(a) No response to tetanizing current (brief impulses)
	(b) Sluggish response to direct current (long stimulus) (reaction of degeneration)

diminished or changed in character, and it may be entirely absent. Under normal conditions, all muscle stimulation occurs through the more excitable nerve fibers. After damage to the nerve supply, both the nerve and the muscle degenerate, and a quick stimulus does not elicit response in either nerve or muscle. A longer and more powerful stimulus, however, will still bring about a response in the muscle. Lack of any response to either muscle or nerve stimulation proves that there is neither conductive nerve tissue nor contractile muscle tissue present. This occurs only in the later stages of peripheral nerve injuries, in poliomyelitis, or in progressive muscular atrophy.

Using the electrical reactions of nerves and muscles as aids in diagnosis, one must always bear in mind that these tests are only part of the evidence, the other part being supplied by the clinical examination of the muscular strength and the reflexes and of the sensory condition of the region affected. A knowledge of the clinical pathology of the central and peripheral nervous system is, therefore, equally essential for the proper interpretation of the findings.

Motor Points. Strong electric stimuli applied to any muscular part of the body will cause disagreeable shocks and muscular jerks in a widespread area. In contrast to this, electrodiagnosis is a delicate and relatively painless procedure that elicits a well-localized muscular response with a minimum amount of current. Every nerve and every muscle, unless deeply covered by other muscles, possesses a small area where it is most easily excited and where a visible contraction can be elicited with a minimum of stimulation. This area is called the motor point. The motor point of a normal muscle is usually located *near the origin* of the muscle belly, where the motor nerve enters the muscle; this area is known as the end-plate zone. In a nerve trunk, the motor point can be found where the position of the nerve is nearest to the skin. There may be several points of maximal irritability in the course of a long nerve.

The topography of motor points was first studied by Erb, and a set of diagrams based upon his studies is shown in Figures 13-1 to 13-5. A set of motor point charts is an indispensable part of the equipment of the beginner; those doing electrical testing should frequently practice the finding of motor points. Even within normal limits, there are individual

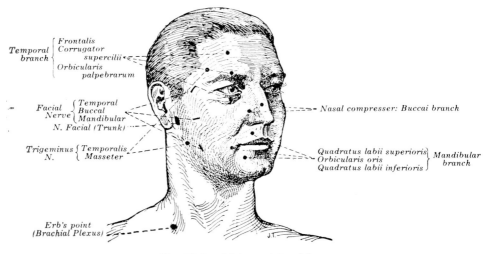

Fig. 13–1.   Motor points of face.

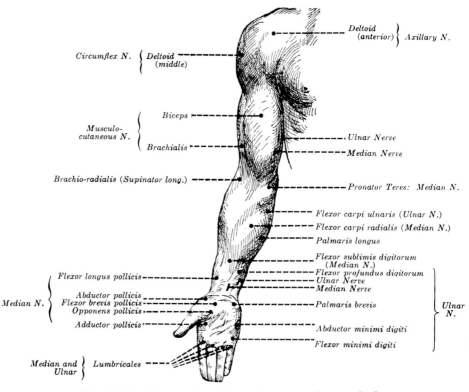

Fig. 13–2.   Motor points of anterior aspect of upper limb.

differences in their location and sensitivity to electric stimulation. In pathological conditions leading to a reaction of degeneration, the motor point of a muscle is displaced distally and the motor points of a nerve disappear entirely.

Apparatus and Accessories. The apparatus for the classical method of testing by tetanizing and direct currents consists of a generator delivering impulses at a frequency of 50 to 200 per sec. and direct current. The true faradic current is rarely used.

There are two accessories for electrodiagnosis: (1) An active or testing electrode, consisting of a small metal disc, covered with several layers of gauze or chamois, and mounted on a handle with an interrupting device (make-and-break key). This electrode serves to concentrate the current over motor points and allows for its make and break. For nerves and small muscles, a disc of about ¾-inch diameter is suitable; for larger muscles, one of 1½ inches in diameter is required. Applying the large disc edgewise also limits the contact surface; too much current crowded into a small electrode causes pain, however. For bipolar testing, two active electrodes are

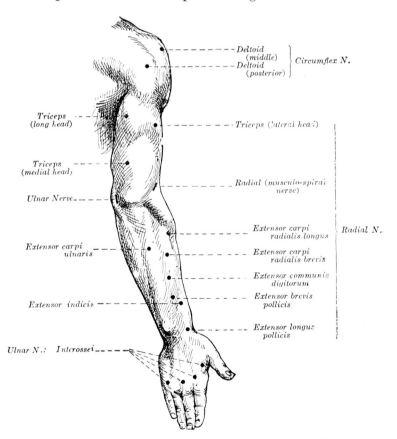

Fig. 13–3. Motor points of posterior aspect of upper limb.

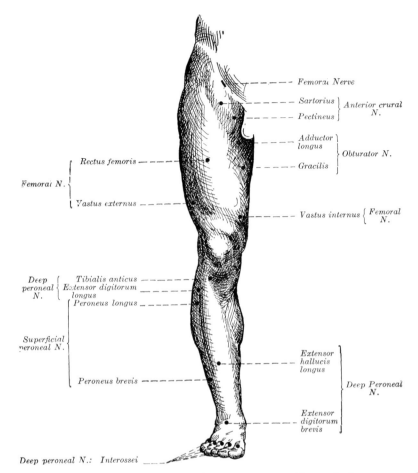

Fig. 13–4. Motor points of anterior aspect of lower limb.

employed. (2) A dispersive electrode, large enough to avoid a current density that may give rise to a painful sensation or contraction under that electrode. A 2 by 4 inch or 3 by 5 inch, or even larger, plate covered with gauze is usually satisfactory.

General Technique. Practical working knowledge in electrodiagnosis must be acquired by testing normal muscles and nerves and thus learning to appreciate the range of normal variations. It is well to start on a muscle or nerve that is easily located and whose response can readily be observed such as the opponens pollicis. A routine for making an electrical examination may be as follows:

The room must be well lighted so that the slightest response of muscles can be observed and warm so as to avoid chilling of the patient.

The patient and the operator should be comfortable so as to avoid undue fatigue. The operator should be able to reach all parts of the appa-

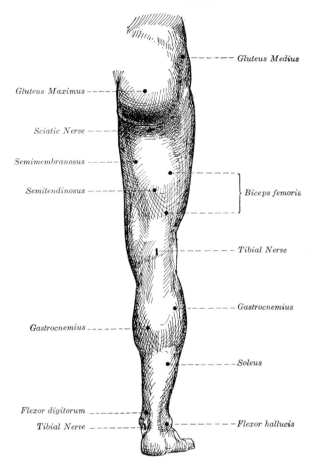

Fig. 13–5.   Motor points of posterior aspect of lower limb.

ratus without changing his position. For testing the upper limb, neck, shoulder, and face, the patient may be seated at a small table, resting his arm on it; the examiner sits at the opposite side of the table. For the examination of the lower limb and the back region, the patient should lie on a table. Support of the parts to be tested is essential for relaxing the muscles.

The area to be examined may be warmed up by a heat lamp, by hot towels, or by immersion in a hot whirlpool bath. The hyperemia produced decreases skin resistance and will also minimize the discomfort of the testing. Electrodes should be well moistened by soaking in hot water. A pinch of table salt added to the water is sufficient to improve its conductivity. A small basin of salt water should be be on hand, and the testing electrode should be frequently soaked in it during the course of a longer test.

6

The routine procedure for testing and treatment is *unipolar testing*. The dispersing electrode is placed over any part of the body with little muscular tissue, such as the chest, the small of the back, or the sacrum. Firm contact is secured by the weight of the patient, by a small sandbag, or by bandaging. The testing or active electrode is placed directly over each motor point to be tested.

With any form of electrical testing, a certain inertia of muscles has to be overcome at first. For this reason, more current is needed at the beginning; after a contraction or two have been elicited, less current will be necessary for a response. It is best first to turn on a current of moderate strength and, on decreasing it gradually, to ascertain the minimum strength, which is just enough to cause response. In paralyzed muscles, often the only response that can be elicited is a slight contraction palpable over the muscle tendon. After the first response, one may shift the testing electrode slightly in order to find a better location of the motor point and thus elicit response with less current. The response of adjoining muscles caused by spreading of electrical impulses is often disturbing. It occurs especially with weak muscles, and under such circumstances experience is required to recognize the slight contractions.

Electrical testing done by experienced operators is rarely painful. Young children may be tested without much crying, once they are coaxed over the preliminaries of their unusual experience.

Difficulties in Testing. As to technical difficulties, it is seldom that the apparatus is out of order. It may happen that after the electrodes have been applied, the galvanic current turned on, and the control advanced, the patient feels no sensation at all and no muscular response occurs. One may note also that the needle of the milliampere meter does not move. If one persists in advancing the current control under such circumstances, the patient may experience a painful shock quite suddenly and the meter needle swings way over. All of this is usually due either to a break in one of the conducting cords or to insufficient moistening of the electrodes. The greater voltage suddenly overcomes the added resistance and rudely shakes the confidence of the patient by the sudden shock. New pad electrodes need more moistening than old ones. The addition of a few pinches of salt to the water helps conductivity. The metal plate underneath the pad is subject to gradual wear by electrolytic corrosion, and the connection for the cord tip soldered on the plate also corrodes in time. For these reasons, as soon as ready-made pad electrodes show signs of trouble, they are best discarded.

Before stating that any muscle shows total lack of response to any electrical stimulation, one should bear in mind that skin resistance, much edema of the tissues, or spreading of current to neighboring muscles may temporarily prevent a response to the galvanic test. In any doubtful case, repeated and careful examination is required.

Bipolar testing consists of placing two small disc electrodes directly over the belly of each muscle to be tested. This furnishes more current density over the testing area and does away with the spreading of excess current to surrounding muscle groups. The bipolar procedure is employed in exceptional cases only, when the muscles are weak and the testing current tends to spread, causing contractions in neighboring muscles. A combination of the two methods can be used. For instance, in testing the intrinsic muscles of the hand, the palm of the opposite hand is laid over the dispersing electrode, and the testing electrode is placed over the interossei on the back of the hand. It is especially useful in radial nerve paralysis.

An accurate record should be kept of the result of electrical testing, and all further tests should be likewise recorded.

The Faradic and Galvanic Test. The faradic and galvanic test was the earliest method of distinguishing between normal and denervated muscle. Although it may be unreliable, it is easily applied and readily available as a simple qualitative screening test. The faradic current, or in modern practice a suitable tetanizing current, applied to a normal muscle or motor nerve elicits a continuous (tetanic) contraction during its entire flow. The galvanic current applied to a normal muscle or motor nerve does not elicit any contraction while flowing steadily, but it causes a brisk single (twitch) contraction whenever it is *suddenly* started or interrupted (made or broken) in a flow of sufficient strength. (See Fig. 13–6.) These contractions are always the result of the *indirect* stimulation of the muscle through the nerve fibers of the motor nerve. Under normal conditions, the nerve fibers are more excitable than the muscle. Only when the motor nerve is in a pathological state and cannot be stimulated does the independent property of contraction of the muscle become evident. Such response, however, is of different character; it is sluggish and wormlike instead of the normally brisk contraction.

The Galvanic Test. The dispersing electrode is connected to the positive and the testing electrode to the negative terminal of the galvanic or direct current supply. Place the testing electrode over the motor point. Advance the rheostat slowly, increasing the current from zero upward. Pressing the key down from time to time, watch for the first visible contraction. With a little practice, one should learn to find the threshold of excitation, i.e., the minimum amount of current necessary for a response. As the testing is being repeated, the needle of the milliammeter will swing out farther and farther with the same rheostat setting. This is due

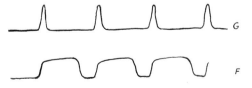

Fig. 13–6. Graph of electric response of muscles. G, single brisk contraction on stimulation with interrupted galvanic current; F, tetanic contraction on stimulation with tetanizing (faradic) current.

to the fact that the repeated passage of the current decreases skin resistance.

The Faradic Test. The dispersing electrode is connected to one binding post of the tetanizing circuit (it makes no difference to which one), and the testing electrode is connected to the other. The active electrode, well moistened, is placed in good contact over the motor point of the muscle or nerve to be tested. Turn on the current, slightly advance the intensity control in the generator, and then press the key of the interrupting handle. The patient will feel a slight stinging sensation under the testing electrode. If the current strength is sufficient and the electrode is in the correct position, a tetanic contraction of the muscle or group of muscles occurs. This contraction will persist while the current flows. After the first response, cut down the current strength to just enough to cause a visible contraction. Also, try, by shifting of the testing electrode, to locate the motor point more accurately. If, by comparison with the normal side, there is more current needed to get a response, note the position of the current strength control (rheostat) on the scale.

Why are two currents necessary for testing? The fact that two kinds of current are used for testing is somewhat bewildering for the beginner.

Motor nerve fibers are stimulated by the make and break of any current or any sudden change in its intensity but do not respond to a current that flows steadily without a change in strength. A standard tetanizing current consists of rapid and short impulses, each impulse having a duration of $\frac{1}{1000}$ second and recurring about 100 times in a second. One stim-

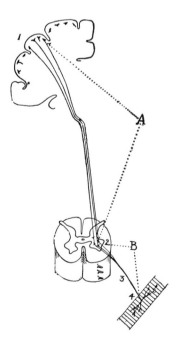

Fig. 13–7.   Diagram of the motor tract. A, Central or upper motor neuron; begins with the psychomotor cells in the cortex (*1*) and continues through the pyramidal tract and the lateral columns of the spinal cord to the terminal arborization in the horns (*2*) of the cord. B, Peripheral or lower motor neuron; it begins with the ganglion cells in the anterior (ventral) horns of the spinal cord (or the motor nuclei in the cerebral nerves) and continues through the peripheral motor nerve (*3*) to the end-plate (*4*) over a muscle. The trophic center of muscles is located in the anterior horn cel's; any lesion above the trophic center results in spastic paralysis, slight atrophy, increased reflexes and absence of RD (reaction of degeneration); a lesion below the trophic center results in flaccid paralysis, marked atrophy, lost reflexes, and development of an RD.

ulus occurring in rapid succession after the other keeps a normal muscle in tetanic contraction during the entire time of flow. This makes observation of the response very easy. The galvanic current, while flowing steadily, furnishes no stimulus for muscular response; only when its flow is suddenly started at sufficient strength or is interrupted while flowing at sufficient strength does muscular response occur. The response to galvanic stimulation occurs in single contractions. It has been estimated that the muscular response to the make and break of the galvanic current through the testing electrode lasts about one-half second.

For ordinary testing, we have individual stimuli of very brief duration—the tetanizing current—and one of relatively long duration—the make of the galvanic current.

THE REACTION OF DEGENERATION

The most important use of the tetanizing and galvanic test occurs in testing for the reaction of degeneration. In the diagnosis and prognosis of lesions of the lower motor neuron of the motor tract (Fig. 13–7), this reaction, as expressed in the terms of the galvanic and faradic test, is still useful, although newer methods give additional information.

If, because of disease or trauma, conduction of impulses through a peripheral nerve (lower motor neuron) has ceased, by either gross anatomical or finer molecular disarrangement of the nerve trunk or the anterior roots or by a lesion in the spinal cord, within 10 days certain well-known changes in the electrical reaction occur. These changes are known as the reaction of degeneration (RD). The anatomical changes consist of the breaking up of the affected nerve trunk and of atrophy and later fatty degeneration of the muscle supplied by it. Consequently, the nerve loses its electric conductivity, and the character of the muscular contraction changes. There is no response to the brief impulses of the tetanizing current and only a sluggish response to galvanism; the latter change is due to the fact that only the muscle fibers immediately under the electrode respond, and the stimulus then passes to the adjoining fibers, in contrast to the immediate response of all muscle fibers when their nerve supply is intact. The importance of the RD lies in the fact that when it is present 10 days after an injury or disease, it indicates changes in nerve and muscle substance that will take considerable time to recover and that in a minority of cases may lead to irreparable damage.

The reaction of degeneration may be full, partial, or absolute (Table 13–2).

Total or Full Reaction of Degeneration.

   (a) The nerve does not respond to either tetanic or galvanic stimulation.

(b) 1. The muscle after about 10 days does not respond to tetanic stimulation.
   2. The muscle responds to galvanic stimulation but demands a greater current strength, and the response is *sluggish* and *slow* (Fig. 13–8).
   3. The motor point is displaced toward the periphery, where the muscle fibers join the tendon (longitudinal reaction).
   4. The formula of polar response often changes, i.e., stimulation from the positive pole elicits an equally prompt or often better response than from the negative pole. This change, however, is not constant.

Partial Reaction of Degeneration.

(a) The nerve shows a decrease of both tetanic and galvanic responses.
(b) The muscle shows
   1. Decrease of tetanic excitability.
   2. Increase of galvanic excitability (this is irregular, most frequently observed in facial muscles).
   3. Slow or even mixed response, but this is not as pronounced as in full RD.
   4. Possible longitudinal reaction and inversion of polar formula.

Many forms of transition may occur between full and partial reaction of degeneration; partial RD may develop into full RD, and both may simultaneously exist not only in the same extremity but also in the same group of muscles, especially in partial paralysis (mixed response).

Absolute Reaction of Degeneration. This term is applicable to cases in which there is absolutely no response to any current in either nerve or muscle. It represents the final stage of a previous full RD with an unfavorable outcome. Electromyographic information is more accurate in determining the extreme degree of paralysis or the complete absence of living muscle fibers.

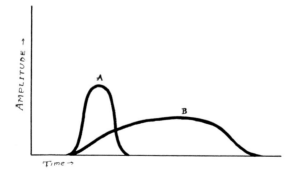

Fig. 13–8. Contrast of galvanic response. A, brisk response in normal muscle. B, slow, sluggish response in degeneration.

Table 13–2. **Electrical Reactions of Muscles and Nerves**

		Tetanizing	*Galvanic*
Normal reaction	{ Muscle { Nerve	Tetanic contraction	Brisk single contraction
Partial RD	{ Muscle { Nerve	Diminished response	{ Diminished response { Sluggish contraction
Full RD	{ Muscle { Nerve	No response	{ No response { Sluggish response
Absolute RD	{ Muscle { Nerve	No response	No response

Course of the Reaction of Degeneration. Whether it is partial or full, the course of the RD always can be divided into three stages:

1. The initial stage lasts from 10 days to 2 weeks. After the first week, the nerve loses all response to tetanic stimulation; the muscles respond feebly or not at all to the tetanic current; galvanic testing, instead of the usual brisk, lightning contractions, elicits only slow and torpid response of the muscles. The average case presents by the end of the second week all signs of the classic full RD.

2. The stage of full RD lasts from a few weeks to a year or more, according to the severity of the lesion.

3. In the final stage, either there is a gradual return of the voluntary function and electrical response, or absolute RD develops and the outcome is definitely unfavorable.

Diagnostic Significance of the RD. The occurrence of the reaction of degeneration signifies a separation—anatomical or physiological—between a muscle and its anterior horn cell and, therefore, may mean any of the following:

1. Complete section of the nerve or root.
2. Compression due to callus.
3. Degeneration of nerve after severe stretch or interstitial hemorrhage and sclerosis.
4. Abolition of function of trophic center in the spinal cord due to anatomical lesion in the anterior horns (poliomyelitis, syringomyelia, etc.).
5. Alteration of the peripheral nerve endings due to toxic lesions (polyneuritis following alcoholism, diphtheria, lead poisoning, and all forms of peripheral toxic neuritis). In the last type of lesion, the RD does not represent all of the changes as in injury of a nerve or in degenerative changes of the spinal cord.

RD is found in the following conditions:

(*a*) Affections of the anterior horn cells of the spinal cord and of the nuclei of the cranial nerves; acute, subacute, and chronic anterior poliomyelitis, spinal forms of progressive muscular atrophy (in contrast to the myopathic muscular atrophy), local affections of the spinal cord if they involve the anterior horns (transverse myelitis, disseminated sclerosis, hematomyelia, new growth, syringomyelia, new growths in the cord). RD occurs in cerebral conditions when the nuclei of the cranial nerves are affected, because these are trophic centers of equal significance to the anterior horn cells. Bulbar paralysis of various kinds results in full RD in the respective cranial nerves and the muscles supplied by them.

(b) Affections of the anterior spinal roots, which may be either primary —due to traumatism—or secondary, due to affections of the spinal meninges (syphilitic) or of the vertebrae (tumors, cancer, tuberculosis, ruptured discs).

(c) Diseases or injuries of the peripheral nerves. Mechanical or chemical injuries alike may cause degenerative changes in peripheral nerves. Injuries to peripheral nerves may result in complete division, partial division (laceration), compression (scar tissue or callus), and simple bruising. The presence of RD serves as an important guide in diagnosis and prognosis, but it cannot determine whether the nerve has been divided or not. Primary inflammation of the nerve, infections, and toxic irritations, as well as inflammations of adjoining tissues, cause various forms of neuritis, classified as toxic (alcohol, lead), infectious (diphtheria, typhoid, influenza), and idiopathic (polyneuritis).

Functional and hysterical paralyses and paralyses of cerebral origin are never accompanied by important disturbances of the electrical reactions. At most, there is slight electrical hyperexcitability, while in the later stages there is usually hypoexcitability from muscular atrophy. *Therefore, the absence of RD may serve as important evidence in determining malingering or functional paralysis* and differentiating them from other conditions.

Table 13–3 gives the summary of the diagnostic significance of the changes in the electrical reaction in pathological conditions.

Prognostic Significance of the RD. The presence of a full RD after the initial stage permits us to state that the seat of a lesion accompanied by paralysis is in the lower motor neuron, the anterior horn cells, the anterior spinal roots, or the peripheral nerve. It does not permit any more accurate location.

It also denotes the severity of a lesion and the fact that it is an organic one because of the marked pathological changes upon which it is based. It has no relation whatever to the etiology of the lesion, because trauma as well as inflammation and new growth can produce RD.

The chief significance of the reaction of degeneration is that it indicates changes in nerve and muscle substance that will take considerable time— months, at least—for recovery. The existence of an RD by no means indicates irreparable damage. It is only a stage of reaction and not a permanent phenomenon, because the lesion may gradually improve and full res-

Table 13–3. **Diagnostic Significance of Changes in Electrical Reactions**

Increased response	Recent hemiplegia, first days of nerve injuries, tetany, spasmophilia, chorea, initial stages of spinal cord diseases
Decreased response	Advanced hemiplegia, tabes, paralysis agitans, later stages of spinal cord diseases, muscle atrophy due to disuse in arthritis, myositis, chronic disabling disease
Reaction of degeneration (full or partial)	*Brain*
	Lesion of bulbar nucleus / Compression of intracranial nerve trunks — Labioglossopharyngeal paralysis, softening of centers, tumors, hemorrhage of centers
	Spinal Cord
	Lesions of anterior horns — Acute: infantile paralysis, acute anterior poliomyelitis of adults / Subacute: amyotrophic lateral sclerosis
	Lesions of cord, including anterior horns — Syringomyelia, hematomyelia, transverse myelitis
	Compression of nerve trunks in spinal canal or in spinal origin — Pachymeningitis, tumors, fractures, dislocations, ruptured discs
	Peripheral Nerve Trunks
	Traumatic lesions — Section, compression, elongation, concussion
	Toxic neuritis — Alcohol, lead, diabetes, focal infections, etc.
	Infectious neuritis — Typhoid, syphilis, influenza, tuberculosis, polyneuritis
	Neuritis (? viral) — Facial paralysis
Absolute RD (no response at all)	End stages of progressive muscle atrophy / Long-standing peripheral nerve injuries or old poliomyelitis

toration may occur (axonotmesis). On the other hand, if the lesion of the lower neuron is not arrested, the muscles will become fully atrophied and absolute RD follows, and all response to electrical stimulation ceases (neurotmesis).

The presence of a partial reaction of degeneration shows that changes have occurred in the terminal muscular branches of some of the nerves, while others have remained approximately normal. The latter have, therefore, retained their electrical excitability. A partial reaction of degeneration always permits a more favorable prognosis than a full reaction of degeneration. It also indicates the necessity of continued observation and the repetition of the electrical tests.

The absence of reaction of degeneration allows the conclusion that no gross anatomical changes are present in the nerve anywhere and that one may expect an early recovery, possibly in 3 or 4 weeks (neurapraxia).

The prognosis based on electrical testing is of particular value in such rather frequent types of paralysis as facial paralysis, paralysis of limbs due to pressure (wrist-drop after sleeping with arm under head), and infantile paralysis. Testing in these conditions, about 10 days after onset, enables one to differentiate between mild, moderately severe, and severe cases. When there is no RD, there is usually complete recovery in 2 to 4 weeks (neurapraxia); if there is partial RD present, recovery may take 6 to 12 weeks; if complete RD is found, recovery will take at least 3 to 12 months (axonotmesis). In organic spinal affections, as well as in peripheral toxic neuritis, no definite prognosis can be made on the basis of partial or full RD alone because it may represent only a transitional stage in an otherwise progressive and incurable condition. In peripheral nerve injuries, the test is less reliable and has no real value in prognosis.

Testing for the Reaction of Degeneration. The patient is prepared as described previously. A motor point chart is an indispensable aid for beginners (see Figs. 13–1 to 13–5).

The usual plan of testing is as follows:

1. Testing with the direct current (*a*) nerve and (*b*) muscles.
2. Testing with the tetanizing current (*a*) nerve and (*b*) muscles.

Beginners should remember in testing one-sided lesions to begin on the normal side for comparison and for easier finding of the motor points. They should also bear in mind that in RD motor points of muscles are displaced toward the periphery and motor points of affected nerves are lost altogether. It is the rule to begin with the galvanic test because it is more comfortable and permits the location of motor points with less current. Once the motor points have been found, the testing electrode may be left in position and the tetanizing test can be done with less pain.

Before commencing electrical testing, one should always endeavor to get an idea of the active voluntary muscular strength present. Muscles capable of active contraction almost always respond to tetanic stimulation. Testing for skin sensation gives a lead in case of mixed nerve involvements. For instance, anesthesia over part of the deltoid area points to paralysis of the circumflex nerve.

The Polar Formula. We have seen in the section on electrotonus in Chapter 12 that the order in which muscular contraction appears in normal muscles is presented as CCC→ACC→AOC→COC, signifying that cathodal closing (the make of the current with the negative pole) excites contraction with the least amount of current; more current is needed for anodal closing and still more for the anodal opening, and most for the cathodal opening contractions. It has been proven by modern investigators that at the make of the current, stimulation occurs chiefly at the negative pole, and at the break of the current, at the positive pole. The generally accepted view is that at the make (closing) of the current, the negative pole alone is active and at the break (opening), only the positive pole is active.

In ordinary clinical testing practice, one may disregard the polar formula; galvanic testing should always be done with the negative pole as the active pole and with the "make" of the current.

Diagnostic Limitations. The presence of an RD may be a deciding factor in diagnosis, but it is not infallible. It must always be considered in conjunction with other clinical evidence and electromyography. For instance, in both anterior poliomyelitis and peripheral nerve lesion, flaccid paralysis and rapid muscle wasting occur and the typical reaction of degeneration develops. In poliomyelitis there is no sensory change, because only the motor cells of the anterior horn are out of function, while in peripheral nerve lesions, since the sensory fibers are included in the common nerve cord, there are always definite sensory changes. The distribution of paralysis in poliomyelitis is irregularly located in the various muscles (with some well-known sites of predilection) and does not correspond with any particular peripheral nerve.

Another example of the difficulty of making a diagnosis on the basis of nerve tests alone is multiple injuries of the extremities, especially of the forearm. Extensive scar formations and adhesions due to longitudinal incisions or multiple infectious processes result in a loss of response of several muscles, thus imitating a nerve lesion. A nerve lesion might also be aggravated by or appear more extensive because of the coexistence of tendons bound down by adhesions. Electrical testing without a thorough clinical examination in paralysis of traumatic origin cannot determine whether the paralysis is caused by the original trauma or is secondary to contracting scars or pressure of callus. The possibility of a coincident systemic infection must also be borne in mind.

OTHER CHANGES IN ELECTRICAL REACTIONS

Increased Excitability. Increased excitability to electrical stimulation occurs in pathological conditions of the nervous system where there exists a state of irritation of the brain centers or where the brain has lost its inhibitory influence upon the peripheral nerve tracts. Recent hemiplegia, early stages of brain tumor, first stages of peripheral nerve injuries, and neuritis may be characterized by increased excitability. In tetany, spasmophilia, chorea minor, and many other rare diseases, the same condition prevails. Increased irritability, however, is of little diagnostic value; it might aid in a differential diagnosis between tetanus and hysterical spasms; in the latter, a decreased excitability is the rule.

Diminished Excitability. Diminished excitability is much more frequent and occurs in three groups of conditions:

1. In muscular lesions following continued inactivity; in such events, clinical findings are atrophy, decrease of muscular strength and decrease

of the reflexes. Prolonged immobilization after fractures or joint affections is a frequent cause of electrical hypoexcitability, as shown in the atrophy of the deltoid after shoulder lesions and of the quadriceps after injuries to the knee. Electrical testing helps to differentiate this condition from the atrophy following true neuritis, because in the latter affection reaction of degeneration is present. The practical importance of these differences lies in the determination of the appropriate method of treatment. In simple disuse atrophy, as signified by slight hypoexcitability, rhythmic electrical stimulation by the surging tetanizing current may result in prompt improvement. Marked hypoexcitability without qualitative changes (RD) is usually characteristic of primary (myopathic) muscular atrophies, such as progressive muscular dystrophy, myotonia, and polymyositis, while muscular atrophies of spinal origin invariably show the reaction of degeneration due to the involvement of the peripheral neuron if a sufficiently large number of axons have degenerated.

2. In certain lesions of the peripheral neuron that are not sufficiently advanced or are not affecting all fibers of a certain muscle. Early stages of peripheral nerve injuries, chronic poliomyelitis, tract diseases of the spinal cord, and certain forms of toxic neuritis may manifest themselves electrically by hypoexcitability instead of a reaction of degeneration.

3. Lesions of the upper motor neuron when there is no change in the peripheral neuron. Late stages of hemiplegia, tabetic paralysis, myelitis, etc., result in simple hypoexcitability due to muscular inactivity.

Myotonic and Myasthenic Reaction. These reactions are qualitative changes in the electrical response, and both are of specific significance in the diagnosis of two typical but rather rare pathological conditions.

The myotonic reaction is characterized by the fact that on tetanic stimulation the muscles remain in tetanic contraction for some time, as long as twenty seconds, after the stimulus has ceased. This is characteristic of Thomsen's disease (myotonia congenita). (See Figure 13–9.)

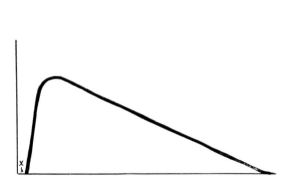

Fig. 13–9. Muscle curve of myotonic reaction; sustained response. *X*, Point of single stimulus.

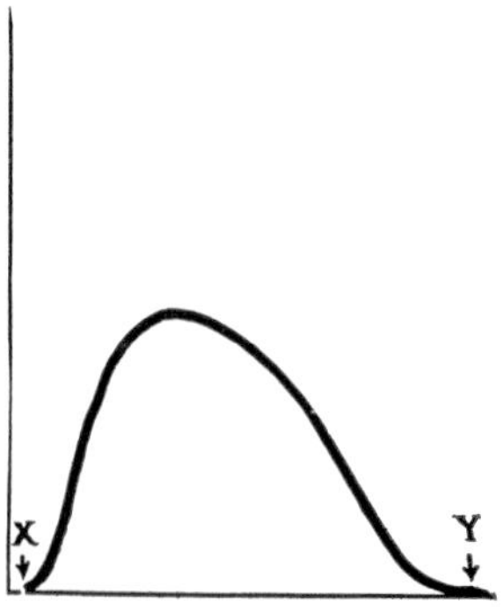

Fig. 13–10. Muscle curve of myasthenic reaction. *X-Y*, time of tetanizing current.

The myasthenic reaction consists of an abnormal exhaustion of muscles; after initial normal response to the tetanic current, subsequent stimulation elicits less and less response, until contractions cease altogether. After a period of rest, response returns and the same process can be repeated. This typical reaction serves to corroborate the diagnosis of myasthenia. (See Figure 13–10.)

NEWER METHODS OF ELECTRODIAGNOSIS

Newer methods overcome the quantitative limitations of the simple faradic and galvanic test through testing by calibrated rectangular wave impulses. These methods allow accurate charting of results, but they require more elaborate and more expensive equipment and much more time for testing.

Testing by Strength-Duration Measurements. To determine the strength-duration relationship of a current producing a threshold contraction, electronic pulse generators are available commercially. They produce the necessary wave forms at appropriately calibrated durations, intensities, and frequencies. A voltmeter and voltage-controlling rheostat are provided so that the threshold voltage may be adjusted and read on the meter for each impulse used.

If an electronic stimulator is used that provides square waves, the duration of each impulse in milliseconds is indicated on a dial of the instrument. The duration of such waves may vary from 100 to 0.01 milliseconds.

Instead of manually making and breaking the current, a frequency of impulses of one per second may be selected, thus avoiding movement of the stimulating electrode.

The technique of testing is similar to that of the ordinary galvanic test. A large dispersing electrode connected to the positive terminal is placed over a remote part of the body and a small ½-inch wet-disc electrode connected to the negative terminal is placed exactly over the motor point to be tested. The stimulus of longest duration is used first, and the voltage or amperage adjusted until a minimal contraction is obtained. A shorter stimulus is next tried and the threshold voltage determined. To get even distribution of points on the curve when recording logarithmically, it is convenient to use values such as 10, 5, 2, 1, 0.5, 0.2, 0.1, and 0.05 milliseconds. It is important to be sure that the highest voltages (400 V) are used only with stimuli of shortest duration to avoid painful shocks.

Some observers have found that a small-bore needle may be inserted into the muscle as the stimulating electrode. This is not painful after the initial prick, and lower voltages may be used, as a just perceptible movement of the needle is taken as the index of response. The reliability of the readings is somewhat enhanced by this technique.

Determination of strength-duration curves is the most accurate clinical method of measuring excitability. Slight changes in both voltage and time factors may be observed that are helpful in detecting evidence of nerve regeneration at an early date. Progressive improvement in the strength-duration curves toward the normal suggests a good prognosis for recovery of function and gives an objective record of progress.

It is at times possible to observe a "break" in the strength-duration curve during nerve regeneration. This is taken to indicate beginning re-innervation of the muscle, and it may appear before other signs of recovery are detectable. A series of strength-duration curves showing degeneration and regeneration in a case of Bell's palsy are seen in Figures 13–11 and 13–12.

The drawbacks of the strength-duration method of testing are that it takes considerably more time and experience than ordinary testing before reliable results are obtained.

Testing by Chronaxie Measurement. Testing for chronaxie is based on the electrophysiological considerations outlined in the preceding chapter. It can be seen by referring to Figure 12–6 that chronaxie is a single point on the strength-duration curve of excitability. Lenman and Ritchie object to any single numerical index because of discontinuities in the strength-duration curve (see Fig. 13–12).

In chronaxie testing, a current intensity of a known contractile effect upon an individual muscle or nerve is applied; the difference in time necessary to get a contraction is the only variable factor; this can be

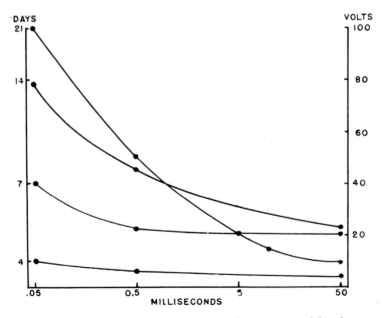

Fig. 13–11. Strength-duration curves during degeneration of facial nerve.

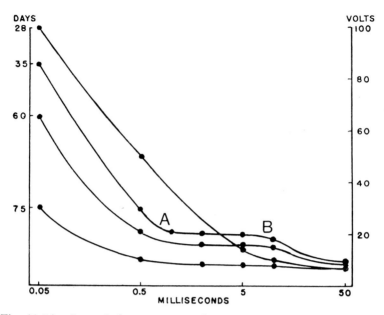

Fig. 13–12.   Strength-duration curves during regeneration of facial nerve. *AB,* Discontinuity in 35-day curve.

accurately observed and recorded. The units of measurement are milliseconds, the range 0.1 msec to 200 msec.

For chronaxie testing, *chronaxie meters* are used. These instruments produce a direct current that serves to determine the rheobase—the minimum amount of current necessary for response in an individual muscle and nerve. A milliammeter on the panelboard gives a reading of this current intensity. The latest machines automatically double the rheobase current intensity when switched to chronaxie from rheobase so that one simply determines the threshold response in milliseconds (Fig. 13–13).

Technique.   The first step in chronaxie testing is to ascertain the weakest current, without regard to its duration, that, when applied to a nerve or muscle, produces the faintest perceptible contraction. This is done by unipolar testing with the direct current of the chronaxie meter, using the negative pole as the active electrode. Rectangular waves in the 500–1,000-msec range may also be used. The testing electrode is placed over the motor point, and the current is allowed to flow at a gradually increasing strength. It is convenient to set the frequency dial to one per second, thus eliminating the manual make and break of the direct current. The ammeter indicates the amount of current flowing, and the intensity required for a minimal response is the rheobase, or the threshold of excitation. Next, with the current increased to read exactly double the rheobase value as observed on the meter and with the testing electrode on the same point, one varies the duration of the rectangular wave impulses.

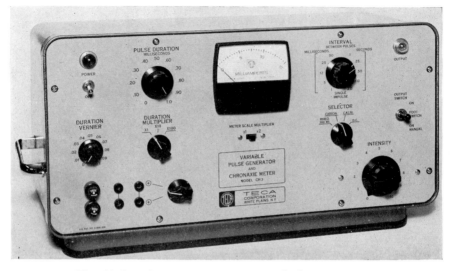

Fig. 13–13.   Square-wave generator and chronaxie meter.
(Courtesy of Teca Corporation.)

By successive trials, one arrives at the wave duration just sufficient to produce a contraction equal to that obtained with the rheobase. This is the
value of the chronaxie. This is measured in units of time because it refers
to the duration of the square wave impulse in milliseconds.

The advantage of chronaxie meters is that as long as the position of the
testing electrode is unchanged, the chronaxie is not influenced by the
skin resistance and the position of the muscle; this allows more accurate
testing and recording.

When the motor nerve of a muscle has undergone degeneration, the
muscle also degenerates, and we find certain alterations in its chronaxie.
For some time after section of the motor nerve, the chronaxie of nerve
and muscle remains unaltered; this period may last a week or 10 days.
After this, the chronaxie becomes very high: 20 to 100 times the normal
amount.

Chronaxie testing furnishes constant values for the purposes of accurate
charting. It has been criticized by physiologists as a measure of excitability, because of its arbitrary and empirical character and because the
type, shape, and position of electrodes alter the results.

ELECTROMYOGRAPHY

Clinical Electromyography.   Clinical electromyography consists of recording potentials of extremely low voltage by inserting needle electrodes
into skeletal muscles. The electrical activity is displayed on a cathode-
ray oscilloscope and played over a loudspeaker for visual and auditory

analysis. Normal resting muscles show electrical silence, but during voluntary contraction, motor unit action potentials appear.

In diseases affecting the motor unit, the resting muscle may show abnormal action potential forms, while the contracting muscle may show various abnormal motor unit patterns. An abnormal electromyogram may indicate whether the lower motor neuron or muscle fiber is the site of the lesion, whether any interruption of the lower motor neuron function is complete or partial, and where it is localized.

Apparatus. The electromyograph consists of electrodes, an amplifier, a cathode-ray oscilloscope, a loudspeaker, and a stimulator. The electrodes may be monopolar or concentric (coaxial) needles. Variations in electrical potentials are amplified from microvolts to volts and are displayed on the screen of the oscilloscope. On occasion, the wave forms producing characteristic sounds may help in identifying variations of the

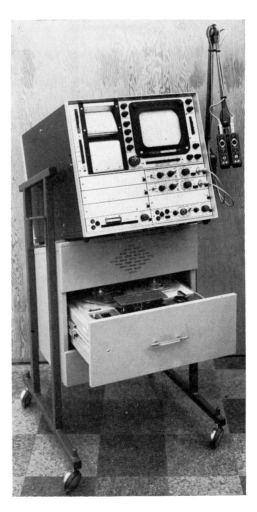

Fig. 13–14. Direct-reading electromyograph. (Courtesy of Teca Corporation.)

action potentials. A permanent record may be made by photographing the trace on the oscilloscope, by storing it on a magnetic tape, or by direct recording on paper (Fig. 13–14).

Action Potentials. *The motor unit* consists of a single anterior horn cell, the axon, and all the muscle fibers innervated by its branches. There may be from 10–20 to 900 or more muscle fibers in a single motor unit. The eye and facial muscles have only a few fibers in each motor unit, while the limb muscles may have units of many fibers.

When the muscle fibers of a motor unit are activated, all the muscle fibers that are innervated by its branches contract together and their tiny action potentials combine to produce the larger action potential of the motor unit. At rest, the motor units of normally innervated muscle show electrical silence. During a weak voluntary contraction, a single motor unit may be active and show a rhythmic volley at a rate of five to ten potentials per second. If the voluntary effort is increased, the motor unit may increase its rate to 40 per second and other motor units may be recruited. During an increased strength of contraction, each motor unit acts rhythmically and independently. Many motor units are active during a strong contraction and display an "interference pattern" on the screen. Motor unit action potentials are usually diphasic or triphasic waves with a duration of 3 to 15 milliseconds and an amplitude of 100 to 4000 microvolts (4 millivolts). A normal electromyogram is obtained in disuse atrophy and in physiological hypertrophy of muscle. In upper motor neuron disease, potentials of motor unit activity reflect the degree of paralysis of a muscle only by a diminished electrical response.

Fibrillation Potentials. Normally, the healthy muscle fibers contract when they are activated by neurons so that only motor unit action potentials are seen. In neuromuscular disease, single muscle fibers may contract spontaneously, and they may be recognized by the appearance of action potentials of single muscle fibers called *fibrillations.* Action potentials cannot be recorded from a relaxed normal voluntary muscle, although they are aroused momentarily during insertion of the needle electrode. On the other hand, electrical activity of denervated muscle does occur in the form of fibrillation potentials, which are of two types: (1) potentials aroused by needle insertion and (2) spontaneous potentials that repeat themselves irregularly while the needle is stationary in the muscle. Both types consist of monophasic or diphasic spikes with initial positive deflections lasting 1–2 milliseconds or less and having amplitudes of 20–100 microvolts. They usually repeat 2–10 times per second and are heard as sharp clicks. Fibrillations of denervated muscle appear from 10 to 16 days after a lesion leading to denervation and may keep up for many months. In the course of reinnervation of a muscle, there is, at first, a decrease in the number of fibrillation action potentials seen. Several days later, motor unit action potentials, some of which are small and polyphasic (nascent) appear. Since such potentials can be recorded only after reinnervation of a muscle, they are of distinct diagnostic value. They cause a harsh sound in the loudspeaker. The interval between the first appearance of voluntary action potentials and detectable functional contraction varies from two weeks in simple compression (neurapraxia) to six months or more in severe lesions (axonotmesis).

Positive sharp wave potentials are of longer duration than fibrillation potentials and are also seen in denervated muscles. They occur as a sharp positive deflection with a prolonged negative phase. Needle insertion or electrode movement brings them out, frequently accompanied by fibrillation potentials. Their origin is not known, but they probably represent the discharge of single muscle fibers or small groups of muscle fibers. (See Fig. 13–15.)

Fasciculations represent spontaneous contractions of motor units or groups of muscle fibers. They may occur normally or in degenerative

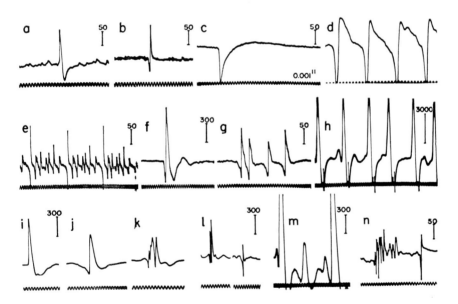

Fig. 13–15. Action potentials in electromyography: (*a*) end-plate noise (small negative deflections) and an associated muscle fiber spike from normal muscle; (*b*) fibrillation potential and (*c*) positive wave from denervated muscle; (*d*) high-frequency discharge in myotonia; (*e*) bizarre repetitive discharge; (*f*) fasciculation potential, single discharge; (*g*) fasciculation potential, repetitive or grouped discharge; (*h*) synchronized repetitive discharge in muscle cramp; (*i*) diphasic, (*j*) triphasic and (*k*) polyphasic motor unit action potentials from normal muscle; (*l*) short-duration motor unit action potentials in progressive muscular dystrophy; (*m*) large motor unit action potentials in progressive muscular atrophy; (*n*) highly polyphasic motor unit action potential and short-duration motor unit action potential during reinnervation. Calibration scales are in microvolts. All time scales are 1,000 cycles per second. An upward deflection indicates a change of potential in the negative direction at the needle electrode. (Reprinted with permission from Lambert, E. H. Chapter 16, p. 276. *In* Mayo Clinic, *Clinical Examinations in Neurology,* 3d ed. W. B. Saunders Co., Philadelphia, 1971.)

disease of the anterior horn cell, as in amyotrophic lateral sclerosis and poliomyelitis. It is important to distinguish the benign fasciculation from that associated with anterior horn cell disease. They are also seen occurring repetitively and may be found with irritative or compression lesions of the lower motor neuron (such as nerve root compression and carpal tunnel syndrome) or in metabolic disorders (tetany, uremia, thyrotoxicosis). Fasciculations by themselves are not evidence of degeneration of the lower motor neuron, but with fibrillation potentials, degeneration can be diagnosed.

Polyphasic potentials may occur abnormally with more complexity and in greater numbers in three conditions: (1) primary muscle disease such as progressive muscular dystrophy, polymyositis, and myasthenia gravis; (2) degenerative disease of lower motor neuron, particularly of the motor cells as in amyotrophic lateral sclerosis; and (3) reinnervation of muscle following nerve injury or neuritis.

Electromyography makes possible detection of minimal degrees of lower motor neuron denervation, direct examination of inaccessible muscles, and the recording of earliest signs of motor nerve regeneration. It is a more delicate method of gauging minimal degrees of lower motor neuron interruption and recovery than methods that depend on electric reactions, but it is of less value from the quantitative point of view.

Watkins has shown the value of electromyography in differential diagnosis. This is particularly true in the case of tremors and muscular fasciculations and fibrillations. Experience has shown that the tremor associated with Parkinson's disease has a characteristic frequency of about 6 per second, which is easily distinguished on the electromyogram from all other tremors such as may occur with hyperthyroidism or hysteria (Fig. 13–16). Visible fasciculation and fibrillation of muscles is a recog-

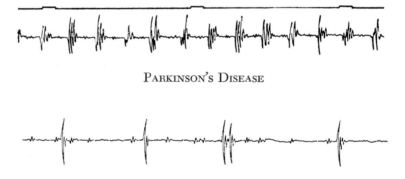

PARKINSON'S DISEASE

PROGRESSIVE MUSCULAR ATROPHY

Fig. 13–16. Electromyogram with skin electrodes of tremor in Parkinson's disease and of fasciculation in progressive muscular atrophy. Time interval, 1 second on upper signal.

nized essential point in the diagnosis of progressive muscular atrophy and amyotrophic lateral sclerosis. The electromyographic recording of these has a characteristic appearance, and at times these discharges may be picked up by this method when not observed clinically. The degree of spontaneous electrical activity is thought to be of prognostic significance.

Electromyographic recordings from muscles have proven to be of value in searching for evidence of nerve root irritation and damage as caused by protruding or ruptured cervical or lumbar intervertebral discs or for damage to the nucleus pulposus itself. The significant finding is the presence of fibrillations of denervation in muscles whose motor nerve root supply has been affected.

Electromyograms are also helpful in the differential diagnosis of polymyositis, muscular dystrophy, myotonia congenita, and the myopathies.

Conduction Time. Electromyographic recorders now contain elements to stimulate nerves and to record the muscle response electronically on the cathode ray screen. The electrical stimulus to the nerve sets off a single sweep on the cathode ray screen. These two events may be triggered by the shutter release of a camera directed at the screen. Time elapsed between the stimulus and contraction can thus be measured on a photograph of the cathode ray screen or with a reference marker for direct readout (Fig. 13–17). The most accurate methods utilize a supramaximal stimulus. Two points along the course of the nerve are selected for stimulation. In the case of the ulnar nerve, elbow and wrist levels are used, and the nerve conduction velocity between the two points computed from the skin measurements on the subject. Delayed conduction has been found in infectious polyneuritis (Guillain-Barré syndrome)

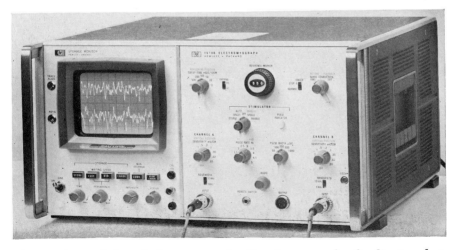

Fig. 13–17. Dual-channel electromyograph with reference marker for direct readout of conduction time. (Courtesy of Hewlett-Packard Medical Electronics Division.)

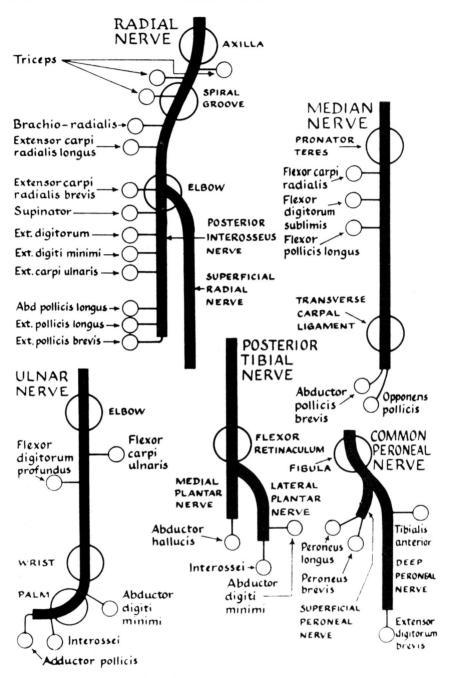

Fig. 13–18. Common sites of nerve compression or injury in five peripheral nerves that are readily accessible to nerve conduction measurements. The large circles indicate the common sites of nerve injury. (From Lenman and Ritchie, 1970; reprinted with permission of J. B. Lippincott Co.)

Table 13-4. *Motor Nerve Conduction Values in Normal Healthy Adults*[a]

Motor Nerve Fibers	Conduction Velocity (Meters per Second)		Distal Latency (Milliseconds)		Distal Recording Distance (cm)	Amplitude (Millivolts)	
	Range	Mean	Range	Mean		Range	Mean
Less than 4 per cent polyphasic motor units							
Ulnar-Hypothenar	50.5-75.0	60.8	1.7-4.3	2.6	6	3.7-21.4	11.2
Median-Thenar	51.2-74.0	60.4	2.6-4.5	3.3	7	4.4-21.0	10.5
Peroneal-Ext.Dig.Br.	46.8-59.2	51.8	2.5-6.0	4.7	8	2.0-13.0	6.0
Tib'al-Abd.Hal.	45.5-58.8	49.8	2.6-6.2	4.8	8	3.0-16.0	8.0
Plantar-Medial Abd.Hal.			2.6-6.2	4.8	8	3.0-16.0	8.0
Plantar-Lateral Abd.Dig.Quinti			2.6-6.5	4.6	8	3.0-16.0	8.0
More than 4 per cent polyphasic motor units							
Ulnar-Hypothenar	45.0-64.0	53.75	2.9-4.7	3.7	6	3.7-21.4	11.2
Median-Thenar	46.0-63.0	54.2	3.0-5.1	3.7	7	4.4-21.0	10.5
Peroneal-Ext.Dig.Br.	40.5-52.6	47.8	3.4-7.3	5.4	8	2.0-13.0	6.0
Tibial-Abd.Hal.	39.5-51.3	46.2	4.5-7.6	6.2	8	3.0-16.0	8.0
Plantar-Medial Abd.Hal.			4.5-7.6	6.2	8	3.0-16.0	8.0
Plantar-Lateral Abd.Dig.Quinti			4.5-7.8	6.4	8	3.0-16.0	8.0

[a] From Marinacci (1968); reprinted with permission.

and compression neuritis from hypertrophic arthritis and in median nerve compression at the carpal tunnel. Normal results are helpful in distinguishing myopathic disorders from the neuritides (Table 13–4). In the past, entrapment phenomena of the peripheral nerves have been difficult diagnostic problems. Not only has the diagnosis of carpal tunnel syndrome been made clearer, but many other entrapment sites have been identified (Fig. 13–18).

Equipment is now available to measure sensory conduction time. The principle involved is that of stimulating, through surface electrodes, the distal portion of peripheral nerves and collecting the conducted impulse proximally. The elapsed time is checked electronically and photographed from the cathode-ray screen, and measurements are made from the photographs. Generally, one has to have knowledge of the range of normal findings for comparison. Such findings are helpful in detecting such sensory neuritides as diabetic neuritis.

Comprehensive texts on electromyography have recently been published. Here one may find the abnormalities present in a variety of lower motor neuron conditions, varying from lumbar disc protrusions to carpal tunnel syndrome. Muscular conditions, such as polymyositis and dystrophy, are also described. There are chapters on varieties of neuritis, including alcoholic, infectious, and allergic syndromes. Adequate discussions are included of more unusual symptoms often of importance in cases of industrial compensation. Some of these texts are listed under Additional Reading, below.

ADDITIONAL READING

Cohen, L. H., and Brumlik, J.: *A Manual of Electroneuromyography.* Hoeber Medical Division, Harper and Row, New York, 1968.

Downie, A. W.: Studies in nerve conduction, pp. 785–812. In J. N. Walton (ed.), *Disorders of Voluntary Muscles.* 2nd ed. Little, Brown and Co., Boston, 1969.

Gilliatt, R. W.: Nerve conduction—motor and sensory. In S. Licht (ed.), *Electromyography.* Licht, New Haven, Conn., 1961.

Goodgold, J., and Eberstein, A.: *Electrodiagnosis of Neuromuscular Diseases.* Williams and Wilkins Co., Baltimore, 1972.

Hodes, R. R., Larrabee, M. C., and German, W.: The human electromyogram in response to nerve stimulation and the conduction velocity of motor axons. Arch. Neurol. Psychiat., *60*:340, 1948.

Lenman, J. A. R., and Ritchie, A. E.: *Clinical Electromyography.* J. B. Lippincott Co., Philadelphia, 1970.

Marinacci, A. A.: *Applied Electromyography.* Lea & Febiger, Philadelphia, 1968.

Scully, H. E., and Basmajian, J. V.: Effect of nerve stimulation on trained motor unit control. Arch. Phys. Med. Rehab., *50*:32, 1969.

Watkins, A. L.: Electromyography in orthopedics. J. Bone Joint Surg., *31-A*:822–830, 1949.

Chapter 14

USE OF LOW-FREQUENCY CURRENTS

Historical. Galvani first observed in 1780 the twitching of the muscles of a frog's leg under the influence of electricity; Volta proved 20 years later that this was due to the sudden "make" of the current flow in an electric cell. The induction or faradic coil was discovered by Faraday in 1831; Duchenne in 1855 described its application for electric stimulation of muscles. Remak first demonstrated the motor points for accurate electrical testing of muscles. DuBois-Reymond in 1849 formulated the law of electrical muscle and nerve stimulation and first employed the induction coil for muscle stimulation. He also made the first make-and-break key for interrupting an electric current. Bergonie of Bordeaux constructed the first device for general electric muscle stimulation by faradism; Kellogg, of Battle Creek, described the first sinusoidal muscle-stimulating apparatus. The newer methods of electrodiagnosis by rectangular-shaped impulses have led to the employment of newer forms of electrical generators for therapeutic muscle stimulation.

General Considerations. Under the term of currents of low frequency a variety of currents are included. Their common physical characteristics are that their voltage or tension is constantly changing and is quite low—as a rule, there is only a few milliamperes of current flow between the electrodes applied to the body. Their primary physical effect is a sudden change of ionic concentration in the tissues affected; their physiological effect is a stimulation of motor and sensory nerves. The term low frequency relates to a rate of oscillation or frequency below 1,000 per second; in contrast, high-frequency currents with frequency over 100,000 per second do not cause any stimulation of excitable tissues.

The therapeutic importance of low-frequency currents is twofold: (1) They furnish a characteristic procedure known as electrodiagnosis for the recognition of pathological conditions of the motor tract; (2) they furnish means for the stimulation of weak or paralyzed muscles, a form of electrical muscle exercise valuable in the treatment of injuries and diseases.

For a number of years, manufacturers of apparatus have turned out apparatus that provides a bewildering variety of low-frequency currents, and there was no universally accepted terminology. Each apparatus was used primarily for its therapeutic effect. Improvements in the instrument were made more for the comfort of the patient than for the effectiveness of treatment. As the incidence of poliomyelitis diminished and a clearer definition of pathophysiology of nerve injuries was gained through experience with casualties of both war and industrial accidents, there has been less need for an apparatus with an "ideal" current. In recent years the manufacturing situation has improved markedly: the number of labeled low-frequency current varieties is steadily being reduced and the earlier confusing nomenclature gradually simplified.

Physiological Considerations. In order to produce a muscle contraction, a current must have a certain minimal strength, and there must be a certain minimal duration below which a current of minimal strength will not produce a contraction. If the minimal duration is reduced, no contraction will result unless the strength of the current is increased. The chronaxie is the minimal effective duration *time* over which a strength of current previously determined as twice the threshold of intensity must be applied to secure a threshold response. Besides the factors of the exciting agent, the electric current, the state of excitability of the particular nerve or muscle treated must also be taken into consideration. This implies that in order to get an effective response the form and strength of stimulus employed must be adapted to the type and condition of muscle to be influenced.

The chronaxie of normally innervated skeletal muscle is found to be usually less than 1 millisecond. That of denervated muscle is 50 milliseconds or more. Because of the high chronaxie of denervated muscle, it is impossible to cause the muscle to contract if the duration of the individual impulses is significantly shorter than the chronaxie. It is, of course, true that if the intensity is increased sufficiently, denervated muscle can be made to contract with impulses shorter than the chronaxie time, but because sensory nerves are stimulated at the same time, these high-intensity currents are not well tolerated. This explains why the *faradic* current with its brief impulses does not cause a contraction of denervated muscle. The stimulating current, then, must have suitable intensity above the threshold to cause contraction. It must have a duration of individual impulse that corresponds to the chronaxie, and the frequency or number of repetitions per second must also be considered for maximum efficiency. Physiological studies have shown that the normal rate of nerve impulses going to the skeletal muscles causing a tetanic contraction is in the neighborhood of 50 per second. The ideal current for stimulating normal muscle, then, is one whose individual impulses are relatively short, whose frequency is between 50 and 200 per second, and whose intensity is comfortably tolerated. Another factor to be considered is the shape of the individual impulse. A stimulus that reaches its maximum intensity abruptly and then dies away less rapidly (exponentially), is probably the ideal. The rectangular wave form is quite acceptable if the duration of the impulse is suitable for the chronaxie of the tissue being stimulated.

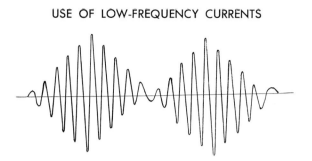

Fig. 14–1. Graph of one variety of surging or modulated alternating current.

The sine wave form of the ordinary alternating house current is not as well tolerated. So much uncomfortable sensory stimulation is produced by this current that the muscular contraction tolerated is not effective.

In stimulating denervated muscle, the same factors of *intensity, duration, wave form,* and *frequency* have to be considered. The duration of the individual impulse must correspond to the chronaxie. The wave form need not be an abrupt increase in current, but rather should be a more slowly rising current. The frequency necessary to produce a sustained contraction is also reduced, being in the neighborhood of 5 to 10 impulses per second, in contrast to over 50 for a normally innervated muscle. The intensity is, of course, adjusted to produce the maximal contraction tolerated by the patient.

In applying these low-frequency currents for producing muscular contractions, the intensity of the current may be manually controlled by turning the rheostat; a surging effect is obtained. (See Fig. 14–1.) If one considers the wave form of the surges, this wave form is often sinusoidal in character, so that this term may be confusing because only the surges are sinusoidal, whereas the individual impulses may have a completely different wave form, such as the *faradic* or square wave. The frequency of the impulses of the stimulating current for a normal muscle may be in the vicinity of 50 per second and for denervated muscle 10 per second, whereas the frequency of the surges might be anywhere from 1 to 30 per minute.

LOW-FREQUENCY APPARATUS

The average generator furnishing low-tension and low-frequency currents should allow modification of both amperage and voltage and should produce surges of regular and variable duration and frequency so as to allow graduated contraction and relaxation in all types of muscular weakness and paralysis (Fig. 14–2). Portable models should allow use at the bedside.

In present practice, chiefly *electronic* types of generators are employed. They utilize vacuum tubes or transistors for rectifying the alternating cur-

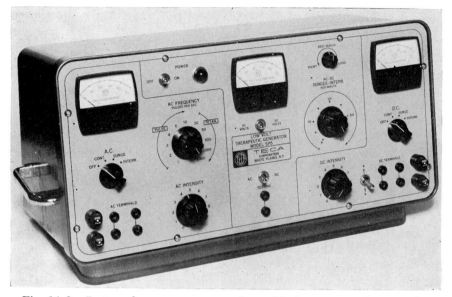

Fig. 14–2. Rectangular-wave generator of variable frequency and surge, plus direct current. (Courtesy of Teca Corporation.)

rent and to change its strength rhythmically; other electronic devices serve to interrupt its flow.

Many modern generators have rectangular wave form, since this form is readily produced at any frequency. These generators allow the operator to select duration of the individual impulse, in some machines anywhere from a tenth of a millisecond to a thousand milliseconds. Frequency is also adjustable to meet the requirements of the muscle being stimulated, varying from 1 to 100 per second or more. These currents are, of course, unidirectional, repetitive, and tetanizing currents when of adequate frequency.

The *faradic current*, produced by a standard faradic coil or by more modern electronic means, consists essentially of a rapid rise and fall of unidirectional (direct) current impulses. The number of impulses ranges from 80 to 100 per second, each lasting about 1 millisecond. The rapid recurrence of these impulses throws and holds a normal muscle in continued tetanic contraction until it becomes exhausted. The interrupting device in the primary circuit of a faradic coil causes a "make and break" in the circuit. The break current in the secondary is much stronger than the make; therefore, from the standpoint of muscle stimulation, the weak "make" part can be disregarded. Hence the effective part of any faradic type of current is essentially an abruptly interrupted unidirectional current (Fig. 14–3).

Motor generators are the older types of low-frequency generators. They produce a variety of low-frequency currents, and additional capacitors or

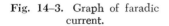

Fig. 14–3. Graph of faradic
current.

choke coils produce a smooth galvanic current. Compared to tube apparatus, motor generators are bulky, complicated, and more expensive;
they have been largely replaced.

Batrow Stimulator. The current produced by this stimulator differs
from all others in its wave form (Fig. 14–4). Extremely high voltages, up
to 45,000 volts, are available, but the duration is extremely low, in the
neighborhood of 7 microseconds. The impulses of this current pass
through a glass tube filled with argon gas at atmospheric pressure, which
allows only the high-voltage component to pass through, completely
blocking the remaining portion of the discharge. This current has the
advantage of producing strong contractions with minimal sensory stimulation in normal muscles. The frequency of pulses is adjustable and may
be varied from one every 2 seconds to 50 per second, producing a tetanic
contraction. (This description of the properties of the Batrow stimulator
is presented purely for its historical value; *it is no longer used.*)

Sensory Stimulators. These are battery-operated pulse generators that
deliver low-frequency impulses for stimulating (afferent) sensory components of peripheral nerves. The stimulators have three controls that
vary (1) the strength of current, (2) the duration of the impulse, and
(3) the frequency of impulses. The patient adjusts the controls to achieve
comfortable stimulation. The duration of the impulse may be varied from
0.05 to 0.5 milliseconds and the frequency from 50 to 150 impulses per
second. The current is regulated to produce sensory stimulation without
muscular contraction.

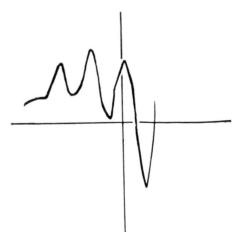

Fig. 14–4. Wave form of Batrow
stimulator discharge. 1 cm = 10 μsec.

This method of treatment is referred to as percutaneous or transcutaneous nerve stimulation. Based on experimental work of Melzack and Wall (1965) and Sweet and Wepsic (1968), the method is gaining in popularity for use in conditions with chronic intractable pain.

STATIC ELECTRICITY

History. Static electricity is the oldest form of electricity used in treatment. After the development of the first frictional electrical machine by Guericke of Magdeburg in 1670 and the Leyden jar by von Kleist in 1745, it was used for the treatment of disorders of the nervous and muscular system by Jallabert, Priest, and Abbé Nollet. Charcot used static sparks at his clinic in Paris for the treatment of nervous conditions. In the United States, W. J. Morton advanced the subject by introducing, in addition to this method, the use of the sustained pulsatory discharge. The

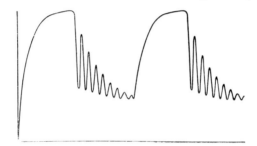

Fig. 14–5.   Graph of pulsatory discharge of static wave current.

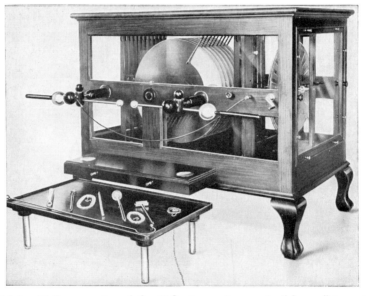

Fig. 14–6.   Static apparatus of the Holtz type. A separate "charger" is contained in the compartment on the right side.

"Morton wave" and other modalities were further developed by the late William Benham Snow of New York.

The use of static electricity reached a peak at the beginning of the present century when the high voltage energy of static machines was used to activate the first roentgen-ray tubes and for the first d'Arsonval high-frequency circuits. The static discharge was a pulsating one at low frequency that resulted in a unidirectional surging current (Fig. 14–5). It was used a great deal in "mysterious" diseases and especially in hysteria. The static apparatus is no longer used. (See Fig. 14–6 for an illustration of this obsolete apparatus.)

RATIONALE OF ELECTRIC MUSCLE EXERCISE

The long-standing controversy over the therapeutic effectiveness of and indications for electric muscle stimulation versus voluntary muscle exercise has been largely cleared up in recent years by numerous laboratory and clinical studies.

In treatment of simple muscle weakness, there can be no argument on the point that voluntary exercise is the most desirable form of activity and that no other form of exercise can have the same physiological value. Yet there are a great many conditions in which natural muscle function is lost or diminished and encouragement of the restoration of function by artificial stimulation not only offers the usual beneficial changes resulting from muscle action but also directly encourages volitional effort on the part of the patient. Regarding the treatment of denervated muscles, it has been shown that electric stimulation does play a role in the success or failure of treatment.

In Muscles with Intact Nerve Supply. When muscles are atonic and wasted from any cause and voluntary exercise is not feasible, so long as the nerve path is intact, the production of painless graduated muscular exercise by electric stimulation reproduces the physical and chemical phenomena connected with normal muscular work. As a result, physiological activity of muscle is restored more rapidly, and all tissues in the neighborhood are benefited by the increased activity. Contracting muscle maintains the circulation of blood and lymph. Acting as an external stimulus to physiological circulatory changes, muscle action not only mechanically assists in prevention of blood and lymph stasis but also lessens the formation of adhesions—perhaps the most frequent cause of long-standing disability after minor injuries.

Muscle Spasm. Normally innervated muscles may be electrically stimulated for relief of painful muscle spasm, particularly if the spasm is not a protective spasm in trauma, such as in fractures or acute arthritis. There are many instances, clinically, of muscle spasm, such as some cases of stiff neck and particularly upper back and low back muscle spasm without significant arthritis, fracture, or ligamentous injury. In many instances, the clinical diagnosis of fibrositis or myositis is made. Stimulation of these muscles in spasm by a suitable tetanizing current may result in marked relief of spasm and relief of pain.

In Denervated Muscles. The main function of every striated muscle is to contract in response to voluntary impulses. A muscle with an injured nerve does not contract voluntarily or reflexly and, being unable to perform its natural function of contraction, tends to revert to noncontractile connective tissue. Since paralyzed muscles are unable to do any active work, it seems self-evident to many clinicians that a method that enables muscles to maintain part of their contractility and their nutrition is a desirable one. Electrical stimulation is the only known means of achieving this goal. The experimental evidence on the benefit of stimulation of denervated muscle is still not completely decisive. It has been quite clearly shown that the atrophy that always follows denervation cannot be prevented. There is some evidence, however, that the rate of development of atrophy may be slowed. Since the circulation of denervated muscle is decreased, it also seems logical that electrical exercise tends to improve circulation. The method of stimulation certainly has considerable bearing on what results might be expected. There is some evidence to suggest that in order to be effective, the stimulating current must produce a sustained contraction of the denervated muscle and probably should be of optimum strength to produce a strong mechanical contraction, possibly against resistance. Some authors have shown it would take at least 10 minutes of stimulation twice a day for each denervated muscle to enjoy optimum effect. The value of 5 to 10 minutes of stimulation three times a week has not been demonstrated. Such stimulation presumably does have some benefit and certainly is often of great psychological value to the patient during the long periods of waiting for nerve regeneration. In the past, experimental clinical studies on the stimulation of denervated muscles in patients with poliomyelitis showed that a great amount of time and expense was necessary to treat such patients, and the evidence was not convincing that it was truly beneficial.

CHOICE OF IDEAL CURRENT FOR STIMULATION

Normally Innervated Muscle. There is a broad latitude in the selection of currents for stimulating healthy muscle. The wave form is not critical, provided there is no slowly progressive intensity to which normal muscle accommodates. Such wave forms are rather difficult to produce and are not generally available commercially. Most commercial generators at present have wave forms that are suitable for stimulating healthy muscle. The critical factor, then, is the frequency of impulses. This should be in the neighborhood of 50 per second or higher, but not over 200. The intensity is individually controlled either manually or mechanically. The only remaining factor is one of comfort to the patient.

The general statement suffices that the current that is most comfortable and causes the least skin irritation while still producing the desired effect is the current of choice.

Denervated Muscle. Many stimulators do not provide an adequate ideal current for stimulating denervated muscle since they provide only a manually controlled make or break of a direct current or a slowly modulated intensity of direct current, sometimes reversing from positive to negative. These currents can not be considered ideal, as they do not have the proper frequency to provide tetanic contraction of the denervated muscle. As previously stated, the tetanus frequency for denervated muscle falls to as low as 5 to 10 per second, and an ideal current, therefore, must have this frequency. In addition, the duration of the individual impulse must be in the neighborhood of the chronaxie of the denervated muscle. Generators that are designed for doing strength-duration curves serve very well for stimulating denervated muscle, as they allow a choice of duration (50 or 100 milliseconds for the denervated muscle) and a choice of frequencies (from 5 to 30 per second) to produce a sustained tetanic contraction. In summary, then, one would like to have available a generator that provides square waves of 50-millisecond duration and frequency of 10 per second. During stages of partial degeneration, one would like to have a generator that provides impulses of 5 to 10 milliseconds and from 10 to 20 impulses per second.

TECHNIQUE OF APPLICATION

Clinical findings on the effects of low-frequency muscle stimulation have made it clear that electric muscle stimulation must be employed in connection with other physical therapeutic agents and general medical treatment and that there is no cut-and-dried formula or prescription as to strength, frequency, etc. for a certain diagnosis. Instead, electric muscle exercise must be prescribed and administered on a strictly individual basis, to conform with the variables in the extent, stage, and individual response of the condition treated.

The comfortable position of the patient and the warming up of the parts to be treated with a heat lamp or hot towels and the preparation of the electrodes is the same as already described in the chapter on Electrodiagnosis. During electrical treatment, the affected limb should be placed so that the weak or paralyzed muscles are relaxed. The physician or therapist must be familiar with the exact location of the motor point, where the muscle normally responds to a minimum of current. The use of testing charts will often save time even for the more experienced operator.

Normal Muscle. Electrical stimulation of muscles may be carried out by three techniques: individual stimulation, bipolar stimulation, and group stimulation. At times, a combination of these three procedures is advisable.

7

Individual Motor Point Stimulation. A stimulus strong enough to bring about a contraction is applied to the motor point of one muscle or to a succession of motor points. A fairly large (at least 3 × 4 inches) moist-pad dispersive electrode is placed upon a part of the body where there are no muscle bellies—the sternum, the spine, or a remote part of the extremity under treatment. An active small-pad electrode—1 inch or less in diameter and preferably with an interrupting key—is placed in good contact with the skin over the middle of the muscle belly, where the motor point is located. The variety of current or current combination expected to be suitable for the condition of the muscle is selected (if not previously prescribed), and while the controls are gradually advanced from the zero position, the response of the muscle is carefully observed. The current strength should be kept down at first to the lowest possible degree compatible with comfort. It must be remembered that with low-tension currents, a considerable amount of skin resistance has to be overcome and that an impulse that at first will not penetrate well enough to cause muscular response may, on being repeated at the same strength after a few seconds, act as a stimulus. For this reason, too rapid shifting of the active electrode must be avoided. Once a muscular contraction is produced, the operator must see to it that it is followed by sufficient relaxation before the next impulse is started. With the double control of current strength and frequency, there should be no difficulty in administering stimulation at the proper intensity and comfort.

The number of contractions to be elicited will depend entirely on the degree of weakness and type of response and may vary from 3 to 10 in a full paralysis to many dozen in a case of simple weakness. The second contraction should be a little stronger than the first, and the third a little stronger yet; subsequent contractions should be about the same strength, their spacing depending on the time it takes the muscle to relax fully before the next stimulus is applied.

Direct Current. The *make and break of the direct or galvanic current*, also known as the interrupted galvanic current, is the simplest means for testing or muscle stimulation when single contractions are desirable. Such a make and break can be accomplished by an interrupting key placed on the electrode held by the operator or by the even simpler method of suddenly making or breaking contact over the skin with the "active" or testing electrode after a suitable amount of direct current has been turned on. In employing the direct or galvanic current for stimulation, one must remember that the "polarity" of the testing electrode has a definite effect on the quantitative response: Under normal conditions, the negative pole is more stimulating. Stimulating muscle by these methods is not very effective therapeutically, as tetanic contractions are not obtained.

Tetanizing Currents. There have been available commercially a number of stimulators for producing tetanic contractions of normally innervated skeletal muscle. The exact wave form was generally not disclosed. Occasionally, the current was falsely labeled as faradic, although it was not produced by an induction coil. These might better have been labeled as tetanizing currents. Intensity of the current was manually controlled or, in some instances, mechanically surged.

To give a normally innervated muscle passive exercise with electrical stimulation, a tetanizing current should be used. One current for this purpose is, of course, the faradic current. The frequency of impulse ranges between 80 to 100 per second and is not measured. Neither is the duration of the individual impulse, which is known to be short and in the neighborhood of the chronaxie of normal muscle. The repetitive character of the faradic current is due to the interrupting device of the primary circuit.

ALTERNATING CURRENT (SINE WAVE OR SINUSOIDAL). The usual A.C. electric currents in this country have a frequency of 60 cycles per second. This frequency is, of course, adequate to produce a tetanic contraction, and this type of current is available on many generators for therapeutic use. As previously mentioned, this is not as well tolerated by the patient because of the strong sensory effects.

Denervated Muscle. In treating denervated muscle, it is essential that the characteristics of the current be selected carefully. The wave form in modern generators is usually rectangular; however, sine waves or triangular impulses are acceptable. Of even greater importance than wave form is the duration of the individual effective impulse. For fully denervated muscle, 50 to 100 milliseconds is satisfactory. If the chronaxie has been measured, a duration equal to the chronaxie of the muscle is used. This may vary between 10 and 100 milliseconds. Another factor of great importance is correct tetanus frequency. On a variable-frequency generator, this can actually be measured and then that point selected for treatment. For fully denervated muscle, this is in the neighborhood of 5 to 10 impulses per second. During the periods of beginning regeneration, the tetanus frequency will increase and is often in the neighborhood of 20 per second, compared to 50 per second in normal muscle. The current strength is, of course, adjusted individually according to the maximum muscle contraction obtainable and the pain tolerance of the individual.

In treating denervated muscles, one must remember that, as a rule, the normal motor point is displaced distally (toward the tendon) and to save time in subsequent treatments, it is advisable to mark with indelible pencil the most effective point of stimulation for each muscle. In the early stage of fully paralyzed muscles, one must be well aware of the danger of overexercising muscle by electricity. Not more than a flicker of the tendon is necessary to prove a successful contraction in a paralyzed muscle. This flicker may not even be visible; it is enough when it is palpable to the trained finger at the insertion of the tendon. It is interesting to note that it may be necessary at first to use a larger amount of current to cause contractions but that after the first one or two contractions, we can elicit response with markedly less current. One can aptly express it by stating that the muscle needs "waking up" at first and then responds more briskly. From 3 to 10 contractions of each muscle are ample at the start, with an increase to the maximum of 30 to 40 effected gradually. A careful operator will very quickly notice that a larger amount of current is needed in a muscle that has been overtired previously.

Bipolar Stimulation. Bipolar stimulation is quite useful in extremely weak muscles; it consists of placing two equal-sized active electrodes at the two ends of a muscle belly. This method is applied only when the muscle is so weak that in monopolar stimulation the current strength necessary for a palpable response causes very strong contraction in the neighboring muscles, which often makes it impossible to observe the response in the affected muscle. With the bipolar technique, the density of current is confined to an area where it is most needed and within a certain limit, this current strength will not stimulate neighboring groups.

Individual muscle stimulation is the method of choice when only a few muscles of an extremity are affected. For example, in radial nerve palsy, this is the preferable method, as it avoids stimulating the normal flexor muscles on the anterior surface of the forearm. This is also true when stimulating the anterior tibialis and toe extensor muscles.

Muscle Group Stimulation. There are several generators available for stimulating groups of muscles (Fig. 14–7). For this purpose, large pads may be strapped to the area, such as along the back or leg muscles. In this instance, the frequency and intensity of the current is controlled by settings on the generator dial. Some generators have bifurcated pads so that a single pad may be strapped to the area without the necessity of applying a dispersive electrode at a distance. One company has designed equipment so that muscle stimulation may be combined with ultrasonic applications. Muscle groups are stimulated, usually with automatically modulated surges and adjustable frequencies. This method of treatment is designed for relief of pain or spasm in normally innervated muscle or for psychological effect.

Duration and Frequency of Treatment. In previous years, overstimulation of weak muscles was much feared, and careful warnings were carried from one text to another that especially in denervated and very weak muscles only a few contractions should be elicited and careful watch should be kept for possible overstimulation. The signs of overstimulation in strength or frequency in any muscle are a slower rate of contraction and relaxation or a well-marked tremor during contraction; several hours after treatment, there may be a feeling of stiffness and pain instead of the usual prolonged feeling of comfort. It was recommended that at the first sign of fatigue, stimulation should be shifted to an adjacent muscle or group of muscles.

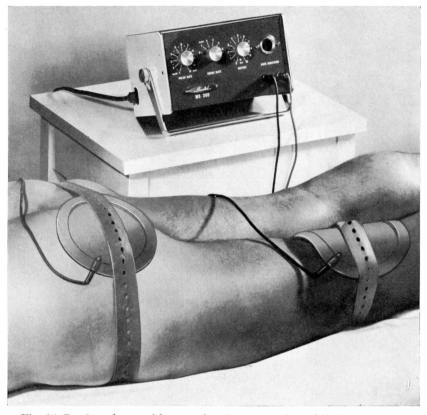

Fig. 14–7. Stimulation of leg muscles. (Courtesy of Burdick Corporation.)

Experimental and clinical work, as well as clinical observation, in re-cent years has brought out some interesting facts regarding the duration and frequency of treatment, as well as the question of load and stretch (tension) during treatment. It has been found that the more frequently a denervated muscle is stimulated, the better is the maintenance of its weight and strength. It also appears that there is an optimal duration of stimulation during which all the benefits of treatment are realized, but if stimulation is continued beyond this point, there is no increase in the beneficial effects. A most important guide is the presence of contractures, which respond to passive exercise.

CLINICAL APPLICATIONS

Nerves of the Upper Limb. *Peripheral Nerve Injuries.* BRACHIAL PLEXUS. In dislocations of the shoulder or stretch-type injuries to the upper limb, including those resulting from motorcycle accidents or occurring during anesthesia, all elements of the brachial plexus may be temporarily in-volved with motor and sensory paralysis. The clinical findings during the first week or 10 days, such as return of sensation and traces of active muscle functioning, are helpful in making a prognosis as to the degree of injury. If there has been no clinical return of either motor or sensory function at the end of 2 weeks, electrodiagnostic testing, including electromyography, is of importance to help determine prognosis. A baseline strength-duration curve may be used at this point for later comparisons. These general statements apply in relation to the discussion of all the individual nerves of the upper and lower extremities to be discussed later. Clinical experience has shown that in the majority of brachial plexus injuries in civilian practice considerable return of function occurred spontaneously. This is also true of birth injuries. Because of the length of the peripheral nerves in a lesion as high as the brachial plexus, regeneration is a long, slow process requiring 2 to 3 years if the lesion has been physiologically complete and degeneration occurs peripherally. One determines the presence or absence of degeneration by electrodiagnostic testing. Many brachial plexus injuries are incomplete and are not severe enough to cause peripheral axon degeneration. This can be determined clinically by the nature of the injury, by the early return of sensory function, or by electrodiagnostic testing. These patients never lose a response to a tetanizing current, although it may be reduced and the chronaxie may be slightly elevated. Such patients may benefit by tetanic motor point stimulation. The current of choice is a tetanizing frequency that is between 50 and 200 impulses per second; the wave form may be rectangular. The frequency of surges can be 5 to 10 per minute on automatically surging instruments or can be manually controlled. In general, the maximum intensity tolerated is used and treatment should be at least once a day in the early stages.

In the more severe cases with peripheral nerve degeneration as determined electrically, one anticipates a long, slow period of recovery. The more proximal muscles are the first to show signs of function; sensory return in general precedes motor return. In these instances, one has to use a current for stimulating denervated muscle, either direct current with manual interruption or long-duration impulses (50 to 100 milliseconds) with a frequency of 10 to 20 impulses per second. All major motor points of the paralyzed muscles are stimulated for 5 to 10 contractions at maximum intensity, preferably once daily or several times a week. Inasmuch as the atrophy of denervation cannot be prevented by electrical stimulation, in general one relies on instruction and supervision in massage and passive exercises to maintain joint and muscle mobility throughout the period of paralysis and assists in muscle re-education as muscle function returns. In a small number of complete brachial plexus lesions, there is actual avulsion of roots from the spinal cord; this can be determined by myelography. Surgical repair of such root lesions has not been successful. Occasionally, the brachial plexus can be mobilized sufficiently for repair if the clavicle is removed.

Upper Cords. The upper portion of the brachial plexus is frequently involved in stretch-type injuries that occur during anesthesia on the operating table or if the arm is maintained in hyperabduction for extended periods of time. In these cases, the involvement is that of the shoulder abductors and rotators, particularly the deltoids, supraspinatus, and infraspinatus, occasionally the teres major and minor, and the latissimus dorsi. These lesions are usually incomplete, and spontaneous recovery occurs. Electrical stimulation of the paralyzed muscles with appropriate current as determined by electrodiagnostic testing is helpful to maintain the courage of the patient. Frequency of treatment is determined more by psychological than physiological rationale. Re-education of the muscles by active exercises is important during the recovery phase to prevent pain and contractures, two most common complications of shoulder paralysis.

Lower Cords. In lesions at this level, the median and ulnar nerves are those chiefly involved so that a paralysis of the hand results. Electrodiagnostic testing is of importance in establishing prognosis. If degeneration is present, as long as 2 to 3 years may be required before function returns. The principles of treatment stated previously apply here.

AXILLARY NERVE. Injuries to this nerve cause paralysis of the deltoid and teres minor muscles. They occur most frequently in relation to shoulder dislocations or fracture dislocations. They are thus not usually accompanied by loss of continuity and do improve spontaneously. The function of physical medicine is to determine the electrodiagnostic abnormalities present and to treat accordingly. In the partial or incomplete degeneration, good results are expected with the simplest of treatment. When degeneration is present, atrophy occurs, and there may be subluxation of the humerus. This should be supported by the use of a sling, and exercise is given to maintain passive range of motion. Abduction or airplane splints are generally not considered necessary or functional. Electrical stimulation if no regeneration takes place is of value chiefly for its psychological benefits. Proper attention must be given to positioning and range of motion. If degeneration occurs and the muscle is denervated, 6 to 18 months may be required before regeneration occurs. In these cases, it has been found that other muscles of the shoulder girdle may take over the function of the deltoid muscle and allow full active abduction of the humerus. For this reason, the exercises should be given to develop these other muscles, particularly the supraspinatus and biceps. Electrical stimulation of the denervated muscle plays a minor role in the therapeutic plan and may be given only as an adjunct to therapy and for testing purposes. There is a small area of skin supplied by the sensory portions of the axillary nerve that is located at the insertion of the deltoid muscle; it is about the size of a half dollar. There may be complete anesthesia or hypesthesia of this area.

SUPRASCAPULAR NERVE. Injury to this nerve usually occurs in conjunction with an axillary nerve paralysis; it frequently is also associated with dislocations of the shoulder. This nerve supplies the supraspinatus and infraspinatus muscles, whose chief function is in rotation of the humerus at the shoulder and assisting the deltoid in abduction. There is no area of sensation recognized on the skin in relation to this nerve.

LONG THORACIC NERVE.   This nerve is usually injured by a depression of the shoulder girdle, as in carrying a heavy pack or load on the shoulder; it is occasionally seen after radical breast surgery or other surgery to the thorax. The serratus magnus muscle is paralyzed, which causes a winging of the scapula. Diagnosis is made by manual muscle examination because of the difficulties in isolating motor points to this muscle, which attaches to the posterior aspects of the scapula and to the ribs. For this reason, electrical stimulation is not satisfactory in therapy; patients with such injuries are advised not to use the arm above waist level. The only muscle that has been found useful in winging of the scapula is the pectoralis muscle. Patients may be taught to hypertrophy this muscle by locking the shoulder in an anterior position, thus preventing winging. This nerve has no sensory component. In those cases of partial lesions, spontaneous recovery occurs in 6 to 12 months. Paralysis is not uncommon after viral infections, especially pneumonia. This nerve is also frequently involved in serum neuritis in patients who are sensitive to horse serum given for prophylaxis against tetanus infection. The prognosis in these instances is thought to be no better than 50 to 75 per cent normal recovery.

MUSCULOCUTANEOUS NERVE.   Stretch-type injuries frequently involve this nerve and cause paralysis of the biceps muscle. As a result, there is weakness of supination of the forearm and elbow flexion. There is a relatively minor skin area of anesthesia on the dorsal medial portion of the forearm in these nerve injuries. Many cases are incomplete, and recovery is spontaneous within a few weeks. If electrodiagnostic testing reveals degeneration of the peripheral nerves, 6 to 9 months may be required for recovery. The use of a sling or other support in 90 degrees of flexion of the forearm is helpful in preventing overstretching of the paralyzed muscle. Attention should also be given to maintaining full supination of the forearm. The same rules for electrotherapy apply here as in brachial plexus injuries.

RADIAL NERVE.   This nerve is frequently injured in fractures of the humerus, especially in the middle and lower thirds; it is also frequently injured by gunshot wounds in the same area. The complete lesion at this level results in a paralysis of the extensor carpi radialis, extensor carpi ulnaris, common finger extensors and the long thumb extensor and abductor. The nerve may be injured by fragments of bone or during open surgery for metallic fixation of humeral fragments, or it may be involved late by callus formation. Electrodiagnostic tests, particularly electromyography, are important in telling the earliest signs of spontaneous regeneration in the complete lesions, as this nerve has very little sensory component on the dorsum of the hand and it is not a reliable index of nerve continuity. The brachioradialis muscle is the one most proximal to a low humeral fracture and should be tested first for signs of regeneration. The wrist should be supported in slight degree of extension, as should the proximal phalanges of the hand, in order to prevent flexion contractures of the wrist and metacarpal phalangeal joints; the thumb must also be abducted and extended. Dynamic splints are usually better than fixed splints, and in any case, splinting should not be constant but should be removed three or four times a day to maintain joint function. If the patient comes in for physical therapy in relation to shoulder function because of the fracture, electrical stimulation may be given to the denervated muscles at the same time. Passive exercise can be given under supervision by the patient himself to maintain wrist and finger mobility. It generally takes as long as 18 months for a nerve to regenerate from the lower third of the humerus to the finger and thumb musculature. The long thumb extensor is the last to return.

Crutch Paralysis. The use of crutches that are too long or are improperly used may cause paralysis of the radial nerve through pressure in the axilla. In this case, the motor branch to the triceps muscle becomes involved first; this, of course, causes weakness of elbow extension, which may result in inability to use crutches. The treatment of this condition is usually to do away with the crutches. The prognosis can be determined by electrodiagnostic testing. Electrical stimulation of the muscle is generally not necessary.

MEDIAN NERVE. This nerve, which is the chief sensory nerve of the hand, may be injured by fractures at the elbow region, by lacerations of the forearm and wrist, and frequently in combination with ulnar nerve injuries, particularly at the wrist. The flexor muscles of the wrist and fingers, as well as the pronators of the forearm and the opponens and lumbrical muscles, are those innervated. A common lesion is the entrapment of the median nerve in the carpal tunnel (carpal tunnel syndrome). This nerve is also frequently involved in a combination of tendon as well as nerve lacerations, which, in fact, complicates the aftercare of such injuries. A period of immobilization and splinting is necessary, depending on the type of surgery required in the repair. Electrodiagnostic tests are helpful in determining whether a lesion is one of complete loss of continuity (neurotmesis) or a simple stretch (axonotmesis). Electromyography is also helpful in determining rate of regeneration of the peripheral portion of the nerve. Electrical stimulation of the denervated muscles following a median nerve injury is not considered of prime importance, more important being proper protection of the suture line through splinting and immobilization of the finger joints and maintenance of thumb in opposition during the period of inactivity. The importance of the sensory component in relation to motor function is frequently seen in median nerve injuries where loss of index finger flexion may be secondary to the loss of sensation present in the median nerve injury. In this instance, electrical stimulation of the flexor muscles to the index finger may establish that there is no lack of motor nerve function but simply loss of control of function through anesthesia of the finger. All physical therapeutic measures involving heat must be used with caution. Manipulation of the thumb to prevent an adduction contracture is useful, together with special splints designed to control proper positioning for opponens function. The same rate of recovery as for other nerves may be expected in the case of median nerve injuries, that is, approximately 2 millimeters per day. Better end results are seen in children than adults. The treatment for carpal tunnel syndrome is surgical decompression.

ULNAR NERVE. This nerve is the chief nerve supply to the intrinsic musculature of the hand; it controls the interossei and lumbricales with the exception of the first lumbrical, which is usually median-innervated, and, of course, the opponens muscle. There is only a minor sensory component of the ulnar nerve, that of the palmar side of the fifth finger and half the ring finger, although the range of sensory distribution in the hand may involve the entire ring finger or omit it entirely. The ulnar nerve may be involved through overgrowth of bone from previous injury or arthritis in the ulnar groove at the elbow or through direct mechanical trauma at the wrist or forearm and occasionally higher up in the axilla. Localization of the site of an ulnar nerve injury is dependent on clinical evaluation, nerve conduction studies, and electromyography, plus x-ray findings. The chief deformity of fingers from ulnar nerve lesions, particularly at the wrist level, is that of hyperextension at the metacarpal phalangeal joints and a tendency to a flat hand, particularly in a combination median and ulnar nerve lesion. Dynamic splints to assist flexion at the metacarpal phalangeal joints are useful, as is mild warmth and instructions in passive and active exercises. Quite a good functional hand is possible in the presence of an ulnar nerve lesion, the chief lack of function being in fine finger dexterity and a tight grip for small objects. Electrotherapy, in general, has little value in the care of these patients.

The sensory component in median and ulnar nerve injuries usually corresponds to a diminished sweating and increased electrical skin resistance. An anesthetic area has high skin resistance, which can be measured on a sensitive ohmmeter designed for this purpose.

Nerves of the Lower Limb. *Lumbosacral Plexus.* Physical therapists are not called upon to treat injuries of the lumbosacral plexus as frequently as those of the upper extremity, as injuries involving this nerve plexus are usually complicated by severe crush injuries to the pelvis. For this reason, only those injuries involving peripheral nerves of the lower limbs will be considered. An exception is the occasional occurrence of laceration of some of the peripheral nerves supplying the gluteal muscles, which may be tested electrically; these muscles are occasionally treated with direct muscle electrical exercise as in any peripheral nerve injury.

Femoral Nerve. The femoral nerve may occasionally be involved by surgery to the hip joint or by direct lacerations in the inguinal region; this, of course, produces paralysis of the quadriceps muscle, which is easily determined clinically. The degree of nerve involvement can be judged by electrodiagnostic testing, as can the rate of regeneration of the nerve either spontaneously or after suture. Sensory impairment of the anterior portion of the knee and leg rarely causes important functional loss. Spontaneous bleeding into the iliopsoas muscle has been known to cause a femoral nerve paralysis, not only in the hemophiliac but also in patients receiving anticoagulant therapy (Benjamin and Nagler, 1973). Recovery usually takes place after 6 to 9 months. In diabetes mellitus, there is also a tendency toward femoral nerve paralysis. The prognosis is good for full functional return.

Obturator Nerve. Penetrating wounds in the region of the adductor muscle may injure the obturator nerve; penetrating wounds in the pelvis may also cause paralysis of the obturator nerve. There is loss of function of the adductor muscle. There is usually little observable functional loss from an adductor muscle paralysis, as is well known when the nerve is purposely crushed in certain cases of spastic paresis of the lower limbs to relieve spasm and contracture. Electrotherapy is consequently not indicated, as it may produce more spasm. Injury to the obturator nerve is occasionally seen after a difficult obstetrical delivery. It may easily go unnoticed and is diagnosed by electromyography. Good recovery is expected after 6 to 8 months.

Sciatic Nerve. This nerve, or its branches, is the one most frequently injured in the lower limb. Lacerations just below the sciatic notch of the pelvis, e.g., from gunshot wounds and outboard motor propellers, may cause injury to the nerve. At this level, the chief loss of function is to the branches of the nerve below the popliteal space; the hamstring muscles supplied by the sciatic nerve are usually innervated from branches arising within the pelvis. Injury to the sciatic nerve at this level can be determined by electrodiagnostic tests of the hamstring muscles.

Tibial Nerve. This nerve gives the motor supply to the posterior calf muscles and the intrinsic muscles of the foot controlling plantar flexion and inversion of the ankle and flexion of the toes. Even more important is the sensory supply of this nerve, as it supplies sensation to the sole of the foot, a weight-bearing area. This nerve may be injured at a level anywhere between the hip and popliteal space with resultant anesthesia and motor paralysis. Recovery after surgical suturing of the nerve is slow because of the great distance from the cell nucleus in the lower segments of the spinal cord that lie within the lower thoracic segments of the vertebral column. A period of at least 2 years must be anticipated before an end result can be expected. Continuous electrotherapeutic treatments cannot be maintained for such a long period of time, so one relies on manual massage and exercises to keep the foot as freely movable as possible passively. The usual electrodiagnostic tests, particularly electromyography, are in order to determine rate of regeneration of the nerve.

Peroneal Nerve. This division of the sciatic nerve supplies the muscles in the anterior compartment of the leg, producing dorsiflexion of the foot and extension of the toes, as well as the peroneal muscle for eversion of the foot. This nerve may be injured from direct pressure as it curves around the fibular head, as from a tight cast; from sitting with crossed legs; or from other mechanical traumata. The sensory component is relatively unimportant, supplying the skin area around the lateral aspects of the ankle and dorsum of the foot and toes. Paralysis of the dorsiflexors results in a dropfoot that should be protected by a dropfoot brace. Electrical stimulation of these muscles is done for testing purposes and to help in muscle re-education during the early stages of regeneration. Injuries at the level of the fibular head require 6 months to a year and a half for recovery and even longer if the injury is at a higher level.

Hemiplegia. The motor paralysis in hemiplegia, whether due to a stroke, brain tumor, or cerebral trauma, is of the upper motor neuron variety. This means that the lower motor neuron connections are intact, and consequently the response to electrical stimulation is normal, with a strong response to the tetanizing currents. Stimulation of the nerves and muscle components peripherally, of course, has no direct effect upon the site of the pathological condition in the brain. The appearance of a normal response to electrical stimulation is often encouraging to the stroke patient, who may be quite depressed, particularly during the early stages of recovery after the general condition has stabilized. Electrical stimulation may at times be useful as an adjunct in motor re-education primarily for the wrist and hand musculature and that of the ankle and foot. The more proximal muscles in general regain their function spontaneously or with the help of exercises. Electrical stimulation of these muscle groups is of little avail. Most patients go through a stage of hyperspasticity of the flexor muscle groups of the upper limb and the plantar flexor groups in the lower limb. Tetanizing currents may be used to stimulate the extensor muscles of the wrist and fingers since it sometimes temporarily reduces the spasticity present; the same thing applies to the dorsiflexors of the ankle and foot. An occasional patient is simply stimulated into greater spasticity and reflex spasms by such electrical stimulation, and in these cases, it should be discontinued. Maximum benefit can usually be obtained after no longer than 2 to 3 weeks of treatments of this type.

Paraplegia. Spinal cord injuries or lesions producing paraplegia usually go through a stage of spinal shock with flail limbs followed by appearance of spasticity. Often there is a troublesome degree of reflex spasm and spasticity. Electrical stimulation is of little therapeutic value and may even make the spasticity worse. Where the level of the lesion is not clear, tests may be done to determine whether the paralysis is of a lower motor neuron variety, as in the case of cauda equina lesions, as compared with upper motor lesions of the spinal cord above the cauda equina. In the latter case, the electrical responses are normal, whereas in cauda equina lesions, definite degenerative reactions are found.

Ruptured Intervertebral Discs. Electrical stimulation in intervertebral disc lesion is useful only when there is an associated motor weakness. In these instances, the electrodiagnostic and prognostic evaluation is helpful, particularly when combined with electromyography.

Multiple Sclerosis. In this condition, the lower motor neuron is intact, and paralyzed muscle groups will respond to electrical stimulation with a tetanizing current. The rationale for such therapy is to aid in muscle re-education through stimulation of the weaker muscle groups. Occasionally, spasticity may be reduced by stimulation of the spastic muscles for 3 to 5 minutes of surging tetanizing currents. Similar or better results are some-times obtained by stimulation of the antagonist of the spastic muscle groups. Such stimulation, although encouraging to the patient, cannot be said to have lasting benefit, as it can have no specific effect upon the mul-tiple sclerotic lesions in the central nervous system.

Poliomyelitis. This disease is truly one of the lower motor neuron, affecting primarily the anterior horn cells. Since the virus tends to attack segmental areas of the spinal cord and since many muscles are innervated by several segments, one finds many muscles with a few intact motor neurons. The rationale of electrotherapy is to stimulate these normally reactive muscles without stimulating the surrounding denervated muscu-lature or, conversely, to stimulate the denervated musculature without causing the normal muscle fibers to contract. Stimulation of the mainly normal fibers is relatively easy, as the usual tetanizing currents can be employed. These treatments, however, are frequently not well tolerated by the patient because of the sensory effect. Although it is possible to stimulate denervated musculature without stimulating the surrounding normal musculature by use of slow sine wave currents with a frequency of 1 to 10 per second, such stimulation requires a great deal of time and has been found not to be worthwhile. One can say, then, that electrical stimulation in poliomyelitis should be confined to stimula-tion of muscle transplants to help develop awareness of the muscle in its new position and occasionally for the purposes of electrodiagnostic test-ing.

Peripheral Neuritis and Neuronitis. Peripheral neuritis of any etiology is, of course, a lesion of the peripheral nerve that causes varying degrees of peripheral motor paralysis as well as sensory changes. Unfortunately, the sensory changes are often in the form of hyperalgesia to such an ex-tent that, even if indicated, electrical stimulation would not be tolerated because of the pain involved. The use of electrical currents, then, is con-fined chiefly to diagnostic purposes.

Myopathy. This term is used in the general sense to indicate any involvement of muscle tissue by known or unknown types of lesions. For example, we would include muscular dystrophy, myotonia congenita, polymyositis, muscle involvement in connective tissue disease, cortisone myopathies, occasionally myopathy due to metastatic cancer, and the myopathy of hyperthyroidism. Inasmuch as these various pathological conditions all involve the muscle itself, there are varying degrees of loss of mechanical contraction upon electrical stimulation, and electrical stimulation is generally thought to be more harmful than beneficial. The response to electrical stimulation and particularly the electromyographic changes are used for diagnostic purposes. In myotonia congenita, the prolonged contraction of muscle after electrical stimulation can be demonstrated and is of specific diagnostic importance. In myasthenia gravis, the muscle weakness is thought to be due to a chemical imbalance in the muscle that is not thought to be influenced by electrical stimulation. It is true that the classical myasthenic reaction can be demonstrated with electrical stimulation, namely, of easy fatigability upon stimulation of muscles.

Parkinson's Syndrome. The rigidity, tremor, disturbance of gait and posture, and other symptoms exhibited in this syndrome are not benefited by electrical stimulation.

Amyotrophic Lateral Sclerosis. This motor system disease involving the pyramidal tracts and the anterior horn cells is progressively degenerative in character, and patients are not benefited by electrical stimulation of the weak muscles.

Syringomyelia. The anterior horn cell may be involved, causing peripheral muscle atrophy and weakness. Such muscles are not benefited by electrical stimulation.

Hysteria. Hysterical paralyses at the present time are seen chiefly in workmen's compensation cases in men. The differential diagnosis usually includes malingering, and a great deal of skill and experience may be required to make a final conclusion. From a therapeutic point of view, electrical stimulation often has much to offer. In most cases, there is an associated sensory loss or anesthesia that does not conform to anatomical dermatomes. Electrical stimulation of the paralyzed muscles, of course, reveals a normal response to the tetanizing currents, and occasionally a single treatment plus suggestion of improvement is all that is necessary to start the patient on the road to recovery. In any event, it has been found best not to continue electrical stimulation longer than about 10 treatment visits unless the therapy is combined with active psychotherapy by a psychiatrist. A clinical impression has been reached that in the male workman, hysteria is associated with a terrifying injury, especially if there is some degree of deficient intellectual functioning. In women, the classical forms of hysteria are seen, including, in addition to anesthesia, bizarre gait disturbances. The latter do not respond well to electrical stimulation.

The types of currents to be used in the treatment of the hysterical patients are those that produce strong muscle contractions of a tetanic character; any tetanizing current with rectangular impulses may be used. It is essential that the current be strong enough to produce a strong muscular contraction, and it is best that it be surged either manually or mechanically.

Summary of Clinical Applications.   Stimulation of muscles with electrical currents of low frequency is a form of passive exercise. The selection of current is primarily dependent upon the state of innervation of the muscle.

Denervated Muscle.   The only method of causing a satisfactory contraction of a denervated muscle is by the properly selected electrical current with impulses of duration corresponding to chronaxie (10 to 100 msec) and with frequency corresponding to the tetanus frequency of denervated muscle (3 to 10 per sec).

Normal Muscle. Muscle with intact functioning lower motor neuron may be effectively stimulated by proper electrical current. Such stimulation is used to exercise weak muscles that may be atrophied from disuse secondary to immobilization for bone or joint disease or injury. Such electrical stimulation may also be used to aid in developing active exercises during muscle re-education.

Relaxation.   Groups of muscles in spasm due to minor injury or secondary to strain, chronic postural fatigue, or arthritic conditions may be stimulated for the purpose of relaxation. This in turn gives relief of pain and freedom of motion. Electrical stimulation is generally combined with some form of local heat and massage plus active exercise, unless there is contraindication to the latter.

Upper Motor Neuron Disease.   Electrical stimulation may be used for relaxation of spastic muscles. Following tetanic stimulation of these muscles, it is often possible to develop greater functioning strength in the antagonist of the previously spastic muscles, thus producing better function of the affected limb. These results are usually only temporary.

Completely paralyzed muscles with intact motor neuron, such as in cases of hemiplegia, may be stimulated as a form of passive exercise to aid in muscle re-education and for psychological effects. No effect can be expected, of course, on the central nervous system lesion from stimulation of the periphery.

Hysteria.   In the hysterical paralysis of limbs, or portions of them, electrical stimulation is often effective. For this purpose, any tetanizing current suitable for normal muscle is satisfactory. Since these patients often have hysterical anesthesia as well, a strong intensity may be applied and is often helpful in bringing back sensation.

ADDITIONAL READING

Benjamin, H. Z., and Nagler, W.: Peripheral nerve damage resulting from local hemorrhage and ischemia. Arch. Phys. Med. Rehab., 54:263, 1973.

Editorial. The value of clinical electrodiagnosis. Ann. Phys. Med., 8:45, 1965.

Johnson, E. W.: Electrodiagnosis, pp. 193–230. In *Handbook of Physical Medicine and Rehabilitation*. W. B. Saunders Co., Philadelphia, 1965.

Leffert, R. D.: Brachial plexus injuries. Orthop. Clin. N. Amer. 1:399, 1970.

Licht, S.: History of electrodiagnosis. In S. Licht (ed.), *Electrodiagnosis and Electromyography*. Licht, New Haven, Conn., 1961.

Melzack, R., and Wall, P. D.: Pain mechanisms: A new theory. Science, 150:971–979, 1965.

Seddon, H.: *Surgical Disorders of the Peripheral Nerves*. Williams & Wilkins Co., Baltimore, 1972. pp. 171–228.

Spinner, M.: *Injuries to the Major Branches of Peripheral Nerves of the Forearm*. W. B. Saunders Co., Philadelphia, 1972.

Sweet, W. H., and Wepsic, J. G.: Treatment of chronic pain by stimulation of primary afferent neuron. Trans. Amer. Neurol. Ass., 93:103–107, 1968.

Wynn Parry, C. B.: Techniques of neuromuscular stimulation and their clinical application, pp. 763–784. In J. N. Walton (ed.), *Disorders of Voluntary Muscles*. 2nd ed. Little, Brown and Co., Boston, 1969.

PART VI

High-Frequency Currents

Chapter 15

BASIC PHYSICS

General Considerations. A high-frequency current may be defined as an alternating current consisting of a million or more oscillations per second. When applied to the human tissues, the extremely short impulse of each oscillation can cause barely any movement of ions, and if it should, this would be immediately nullified by an impulse coming from the opposite direction. Because of the absence of electrochemical reactions, there is no stimulation of sensory and motor nerves, in contrast to all other forms of electricity. Instead, the energy of the rapidly oscillating current is transformed into heat energy along its path.

The production of heat is not a specific property of the high-frequency current, for any electric current, in accordance with Joule's laws, will heat tissues. Low-frequency currents are not suitable for tissue heating because their electrolytic or polarity effects will bring about tissue destruction at any strength that would cause an appreciable heating.

There are three methods of high-frequency tissue heating. The oldest method, now obsolete, is known as long-wave diathermy. It employed oscillations of a frequency of about a million per second and was applied through bare metal electrodes placed in direct contact with the skin or mucous membranes. The present method of short-wave diathermy has replaced long-wave diathermy and employs oscillations from 10 to 100 million per second. It is routinely applied through a spacing of air or rubber. In microwave diathermy, oscillations of some 3,000 million per second are used by focusing a single beam of electromagnetic energy from some distance to the region to be treated. Long-wave diathermy is produced by obsolete spark gap apparatus, and short-wave diathermy as a rule, by tube apparatus, while microwaves are produced by a magnetron oscillator.

The frequency of electromagnetic oscillations sent out by a spark gap or oscillator tube generator is determined by the physical characteristics of the generating circuit. The basic principles of thermionic devices and electromagnetic oscillations have been already presented in Chapters 8 and 9. All electromagnetic waves travel at the speed of light, 186,000 miles or 300,000 kilometers per second in vacuum. The generally accepted view of the propagation of electromagnetic oscillations is that they pro-

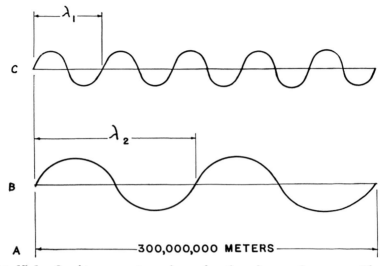

Fig. 15–1. Graphic comparison of wavelength and wave frequency. The base line *A* is a distance over which electromagnetic waves *B* and *C* travel with the same speed (300 million meters per second). They cover the same distance in the same amount of time; the oscillation frequency of the longer waves, *B*, is less than that of the shorter waves, *C*. The shorter the wavelength, the greater is the frequency of oscillations. λ_1 and λ_2 are the wavelengths of the oscillations.

ceed in the form of waves and since all these waves travel at the same speed it is evident that the wavelengths of those of high-frequency oscillation are shorter, as indicated in Figure 15–1. In other words, the higher the frequency of a certain form of electromagnetic energy, the shorter its wavelength.

The electromagnetic waves of short-wave diathermy are generated by the same physical means as those of the short-wave radio band and are, as a matter of fact, identical with them. Hence the necessity for regulations to avoid interference with radio communications. However, for therapeutic purposes, the oscillations produced are not transferred to an "open circuit" through aerial and ground connections but to a "closed" or treatment circuit between which the part to be treated is placed. Actually, the treatment plates, when paired in this manner, form a condenser or capacitor. The part to be treated is introduced into the electric field between the plates; this field conveys regular impulses to the particles of the substance. When these impulses enter the body tissues, they become a high-frequency current.

Microwaves possess optical properties. They can be reflected, refracted, and diffracted, and they can be focused by suitable lenses and reflectors much as can the beam of a searchlight. This permits their use under the name of radar for detecting such objects as ships, airplanes, and the periscopes of submarines. They are absorbed by water and are selectively absorbed by the atmosphere and by the body tissues. They must be conducted from the generator to the applicator by a coaxial cable.

For the differentiation of various electromagnetic waves, a statement of their frequency suffices; this is done to a certain extent in radio broadcasting. In physical therapy, it has become the established custom to describe these forms of energy by stating their wavelength.

The relation of wavelength and frequency in the most frequently employed therapeutic electromagnetic oscillations is as follows:

	Wavelength (approximate)	Frequency
Short-wave diathermy	30 to 3 meters	10 to 100 million cycles per second (10 to 100 megacycles)
Microwave diathermy	1 meter to 10 centimeters	300 to 3,000 million cycles per second (300 to 3,000 megacycles)

Basic Physics of Apparatus. The commercial alternating current serves, as a rule, as the source of all high-frequency currents. In order to produce oscillations of sufficiently high frequency and power to heat the human tissues, two essential changes have to be effected in this current: (1) The voltage must be increased; this is done by transformers and rectifiers. (2) The high-frequency wave must be produced; this is done by an "oscillating circuit," consisting of a capacitor, an inductance, and an oscillating tube in the vacuum-tube apparatus.

We will now discuss some details of the production of electric oscillations, in addition to the basic principles already presented at the end of Chapter 9. The oscillations are produced by the oscillating tubes and are sustained by the inductance, the most essential part of any oscillating circuit. The inductance consists of a solenoid, a coil of copper wire. Such a solenoid offers very little ohmic or "conductive" resistance to the passage of a direct current but offers an enormous "inductive" resistance to the oscillating current that the electrical energy of the capacitor discharges. As a result, instead of a sudden dying out of the electrical charge, the current oscillates back and forth at a frequency determined by the capacitance and the inductance. The other devices in the generating circuit sustain the oscillations (Figs. 15–2 and 15–3).

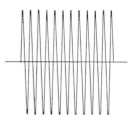

Fig. 15–2.   Graph of oscillations of short-wave diathermy.

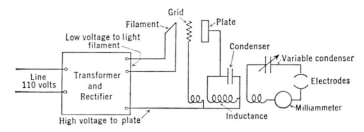

Fig. 15–3. Schematic diagram of vacuum tube oscillator.

The important property of an oscillator circuit is that any desired wavelength may be obtained by suitable variation of the physical characteristics of the circuit. The frequency is determined by the capacity of the circuit, which depends on the surface area and number of plates of the capacitor, and the inductance, which depends on the diameter and number of turns in the coil.

Vacuum-Tube Apparatus. The three principal divisions of the vacuum-tube apparatus are (1) the internal power supply, (2) the oscillator, (3) the resonator or external patient circuit. The details of these circuits and the frequencies produced vary in different types of apparatus. Figure 15–3 schematically illustrates one of the simplest and most typical constructions.

(*a*) The *internal power supply circuit* contains at least two transformers: a step-down transformer to provide a low-voltage alternating current to light the filaments of the oscillator tubes and a step-up transformer to provide a high-voltage direct current for the plates of these tubes. The "rectification" or change of the alternating current into a direct current for the plate is usually produced by rectifier tubes.

(*b*) The *oscillator circuit* produces the high-frequency oscillations. It consists of a grid circuit, one or two oscillator tubes, and a plate circuit. The grid circuit contains a coil and condenser whose values of capacity and inductance have been fixed to determine the frequency desired from the machine. This circuit provides a source of voltage at the grid of the oscillator tubes. This voltage is reversed during each high-frequency cycle. Thus, many millions of times a second the electrical voltage of the tube changes. The plate circuit, or tank circuit, is also made up of capacitance and inductance. These two circuits, being resonant to the same frequency, energize each other to maintain oscillation at their characteristic frequency.

(*c*) The *external patient circuit* also consists of inductance and capacitance. Either or both may be variable in order to "tune" this circuit, but usually the coil is fixed and the capacitor is variable. The tuning device of most short-wave diathermy machines is this variable capacitor. It serves to bring the patient circuit into resonance with the oscillator frequency, just as one resonates a radio set when he tunes in a station. When the capacitor is finely tuned, it allows the maximum transfer of inductive energy from the oscillator to the patient. As one slightly detunes the capacitor, less energy is extracted from the oscillator circuit.

A milliammeter is placed in short-wave apparatus, usually in the plate circuit of the oscillator. It serves primarily as an indicator that electrical energy is passing. The removal of energy from the oscillator to the patient causes a greater current drain, which is noted by a rise in the meter. The meter will also indicate that at a certain position of the capacitor controls— when the patient's circuit is "tuned" to the main oscillator circuit—there is a maximal flow of energy in the treatment field. Since the patient is in the resonator circuit, any movement he makes will alter the capacitance of the patient circuit. This detunes the circuit, and the energy falls off.

The tubes are the heart of the short-wave apparatus, and on their proper function depends the efficient output of the apparatus. Tubes are not made by manufacturers of apparatus but are received by them under a guarantee that they are free from electrical and mechanical defects. Well-made and properly operated tubes have a normal life of from 500 to 1,000 hours. At the end of this period they do not as a rule burn out but rather gradually decrease in output. A defective tube will result in the dropping off in power of the apparatus; it may also cause overheating of another tube in the circuit. A crack in the glass of a tube will result in the admission of air and destruction of the tube. Transistors that eliminate these tube problems are not, as yet, used very much in diathermy apparatus.

Controls of Vacuum Tube Apparatus. The controls and steps in operating the average short-wave diathermy apparatus are as follows:

The main switch or power inlet provides the supply current flow. It serves first for the warming up of the filament (cathode) in the vacuum tubes. It takes a few seconds for this heating. The filament should always be allowed to heat up for several seconds to a minute before the plate voltage is turned on.

The current output control allows the turning on of an increasing amount of supply current to the oscillator tubes according to the amount of energy required by the patient's circuit.

Microwave (Magnetron Tube) Apparatus. Microwave apparatus consists of two principal divisions:

(*a*) *The power supply circuit* provides a high-voltage fully filtered direct current to the oscillator tube. It contains a step-up transformer and a rectifier circuit. In addition, the power section supplies low-voltage alternating current to the filaments of the rectifier tubes and the magnetron oscillator tube.

(*b*) *The magnetron oscillator* is a tube that incorporates a complete oscillator circuit and is capable of generating radio-frequency energy at centimeter wavelengths. The tube is essentially a diode consisting of two elements—the cathode and the anode. Its operation is best described by comparing it to a whistle. If air of sufficient volume and velocity is blown across the cavity of a whistle, a sound will be emitted, the pitch of which is determined by the volume of the cavity. In like manner, a stream of electrons may be passed over a cavity, causing the cavity to become excited at a predetermined frequency determined by the shape and size of the cavity. Utilizing this principle, a series of keyhole-shaped cavities are cut into the anode of the magnetron (the anode itself is cylindrical). The center element of the magnetron is known as the cathode. This cathode is a nickel cylinder coated with barium and strontium oxide that supplies a copious flow of electrons when heated (Fig. 15–4). The usual microwave diathermy magnetron has sixteen identical cavities, all of which oscillate at the same frequency. These circuits are all part of the tube enclosed in a vacuum, so they are not affected by dust, dirt, or humidity. A coaxial cable (Fig. 15–5) is employed for transmitting the energy from the magnetron tube to the applicator device. In order to

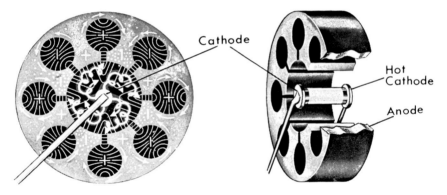

Fig. 15–4. Construction of magnetron oscillator and scheme of electron flow.

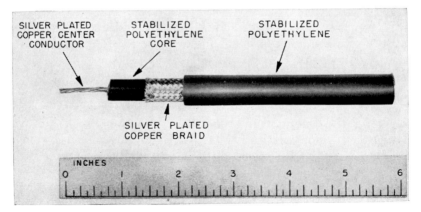

Fig. 15–5. Coaxial cable of magnetron oscillator.

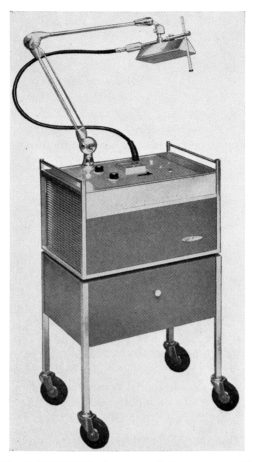

Fig. 15–6. Burdick MW-200 microwave diathermy unit with E director.
(Courtesy of Burdick Corporation.)

apply the energy to the patient, a director is employed (Fig. 15–6). This director is actually an antenna around which a beam-forming plate has been constructed. The director beams the energy toward a given area, eliminating pads, coils, and other electrodes. There is no contact between the patient and the machine. Microwave generators operating in the band from 2400 to 2500 megacycles do not interfere with radio or television.

Controls and Operation. Because of the nature of the generator and the stability of microwave diathermy, there is no "patient circuit" in the apparatus. There is no necessity for tuning microwave equipment at all. The director is actually an antenna, and the patient is independent of the apparatus, simply receiving radiated energy from this antenna. The controls consist of a preheat switch, power switch, power control, and a treatment-timing device.

To operate the equipment, the preheat switch is put in the "on" position, and the preheat indicating light lights up. Another indicator light is used to show when the necessary preheating period is over. The preheat switch merely allows line voltage to enter the equipment, lighting the filaments of the tubes. Until the power light comes on, it is impossible to apply the high voltage to the magnetron oscillator tube. The power switch may now be put in the "on" position and the treatment timer set. Next, the power control is turned clockwise until the desired output is reached, as indicated on the meter. The power level may be adjusted at any time and read on the meter. Upon expiration of the treatment time, the power will automatically shut off, leaving the preheat on and the machine ready for the next treatment. The newer models require no warming-up period.

Radio Interference by Electrical Apparatus. Sparking in the circuit of any household or medical electrical apparatus may cause radio interference. This is minimal in low-voltage apparatus, while with high-voltage and high-frequency apparatus, it may become very annoying, as the electric energy produced can surge back through the power supply into the power line or actually radiate into space as radio waves. In accordance with international agreements, the U.S. Federal Communications Commission has restricted the frequencies of "type-approved" short-wave diathermy apparatus to approximately 22, 11, and $7\frac{1}{2}$ meters wavelength.

Higher frequencies used in short-wave machines radiate efficiently from shorter wires, and therefore a considerable amount of energy may leave the conducting leads. The energy that leaves the wire is more likely to travel far, by virtue of refraction and reflection by the stratospheric Kennelly-Heaviside layer of ionized particles.

It is now known that the great distances spanned by radio waves are due to the reflection of waves by a layer of electrically charged atoms and molecules in the upper atmosphere. A transmitter radiates waves that are bent back by this Kennelly-Heaviside layer toward the earth, where they are again reflected upward. The process of refraction by the ionic layer and reflection by the earth's surface repeats itself all around the earth. The Kennelly-Heaviside layer does not reflect the ultrahigh-frequency waves used in microwave, television, and radar. For this reason, television and radar receivers must be within sight of the transmitting antenna.

Table 15–1. High-Frequency Medical Treatment Methods

	Technique	Effect
Microwave diathermy	Energy beamed through single director	Localized heating
Short-wave diathermy	Electric field heating	Depth heating of all tissues
	Electromagnetic field heating	Heating chiefly vascular tissues

Methods of High-Frequency Treatments. High-frequency currents are applied either for treatment within physiological toleration of tissues—medical high frequency or diathermy—or for destruction of new growths and diseased tissues—surgical diathermy or electrosurgery. Table 15–1 gives a condensed presentation of medical high-frequency methods.

ADDITIONAL READING

Schwan, H. P.: Biophysics of diathermy. In S. Licht (ed.), *Therapeutic Heat and Cold*. 2nd ed. Waverly Press, Baltimore, 1965.
Woodruff, H. C.: *ABC's of Microwaves*. Howard W. Sams and Co., Indianapolis, 1969.

Chapter 16

MEDICAL DIATHERMY

General Considerations. The principal physical effect of high-frequency treatment is the heating of the human tissues. The production of heat is not a specific property of the high-frequency current, for any electrical current, in accordance with Joule's laws, will heat tissues. Low-frequency currents are not suitable for tissue heating because their electrolytic or polarity effects will bring about tissue destruction at any strength that would cause appreciable heating. Radiant sources of heating (heat lamps and infrared generators) as well as conductive sources of heating (hot-water battles and electric pads) produce chiefly superficial heating, as shown by the skin redness due to dilatation of the capillaries. It is also evident that in any "external" heating through the skin, increased circulation and perspiration will tend to disperse some of the heat and preclude deeper penetration. It is, furthermore, difficult, if not impossible, to cause intensive heating of deeper parts by conductive heating without overheating the skin. The experimental proofs of the penetrating heating by diathermy and the clinical results produced by it have established high-frequency tissue heating as an important tissue-heating method in physical medicine.

Experimental Demonstrations. Three classical experiments have been employed with long-wave diathermy apparatus for many years to demonstrate the basic physical effect of a high-frequency current upon conductors and its difference from that of a low-frequency current.

(*a*) Water Experiment. *The high-frequency current exerts no electrolytic or electrochemical effect.* The tips of two conducting cords leading from the terminals are placed about 2 inches apart in a flat vessel containing tap water. Turning on a fair amount of current, the excursion of the meter needle will show passage of the current, but no bubbles appear around either cord tip, no matter how long the current flows. If a few pinches of salt are added to the water, the meter will rise further, showing the passage of more current due to increased conductivity, but there still will be no formation of gas bubbles.

(*b*) Light Bulb Experiment. *The high-frequency current exerts heating effects on the body without causing neuromuscular stimulation.* A person

212

holds a cylindrical electrode in each hand; the base of one cylinder is connected to one terminal of the high-frequency machine, the base of the other to an electric light bulb (socket-testing device). The latter is then connected to the second terminal. As soon as the current is turned on, the lamp lights up, yet the individual through whom the current passes perceives practically no sensation and there is no muscular twitch.

(c) Wrist Experiment. *The maximum heat effect of a high-frequency current occurs along the shortest path of the current, where the density is greatest.* A person grips one cylindrical electrode or the short-wave cable in each hand, holding the wrists straight. With current turned on, more heat is felt in the wrists than the hand or forearm.

THERMAL EFFECT OF DIATHERMY

High-frequency electrical energy extends from electrode to electrode through the human tissues or penetrates deeply into the tissues from a suitable applicator; it has become the standard method for deeper tissue heating in the body. The basic laws for heating of conductors are those known as Joule's laws: (a) The heat produced is directly proportional to the square of the current strength. (b) The heat produced by a given amount of current is directly proportional to the resistance of the conductor. (c) The heat produced is directly proportional to the time during which the current flows. The actual heating of tissues depends on the number of calories supplied to the tissues per second by the high-frequency current. This can be expressed as a power unit: 1 watt equals 0.239 calories per second.

In considering heat distribution in the various parts of the body, the question of heat loss by conduction, radiation, and convection must always be taken into account. In highly vascular organs, such as the lungs, the blood always carries away a considerable amount of heat. The tissue temperature distribution depends on the thermal property of the tissue, i.e., the specific heat and density. It also depends on the thermal conductivity of the tissues, which may vary with time. The temperature distribution is modified by physiological factors such as the temperature of the tissues before the exposure to the diathermy and the changes in blood flow. Usually, the skin surface is relatively cool, while the central or core temperature is warm. As diathermy is applied, an increase in blood flow may occur locally as a result of changes in the tissue temperature. Since the temperature of the blood is usually lower than that of heated tissue, it may act as a cooling agent.

These general principles of heat production and distribution prevail with all methods of diathermy, whereas the passage of current and the distribution of heating vary somewhat with the different techniques.

Heating in the Electric Field. Currents of a frequency of ten million or more oscillations per second, as employed in short-wave diathermy, can be induced more readily in substances that are nonconductive than can a current of lower frequency. These higher-frequency oscillations can therefore be conveyed to the body through a layer of air, insulating pad, or an insulated cable. This allows a more flexible and often more convenient and safer technique. There is no need to ensure good contact, as with metal contact plates; uneven surfaces can be treated; and the problems of edge effect are greatly reduced.

It is the physical characteristic of electric oscillations of very high frequency that in a capacitor arrangement with conductive tissue placed between two electrodes, part of the electric charge will pass as a conduction current and part of it as a so-called "current of capacity." It has been found experimentally that the higher the frequency of the current applied, the greater is the "capacitative" component and the smaller is the conductive current component. It is therefore claimed that because of the dielectric property of some of the ordinarily poorly conductive tissues, a very high-frequency current may cause effective heating in regions that would otherwise be more or less inaccessible to a purely conductive current. It has been shown that short-wave diathermy causes significant increase in temperature in thigh muscles of man; in the liver, spleen, lung, and kidney of anesthetized dogs; and in cerebrospinal fluid in man.

Heating in the Electromagnetic Field. A flexible heat-insulated cable in the form of a coil or loop is wound around a limb or is placed in the form of a pancake over part of the body. A high-frequency current traversing such a coil creates a magnetic field, and in conductive substances placed inside this field, induced currents known as *eddy currents* will arise; these flow in a direction opposite to that of the changing current in the coil. If of sufficient strength, the eddy current generates heat in such conductive substances as the soft tissues of the human body.

The eddy currents induced in the more conductive materials will be more intense, and, therefore, the generation of heat per unit of time will be greater in these than in the less conductive materials. Obviously, if a body composed of materials of different electrical conductivities, such as the tissues of the human body, is placed within the field, the intensity of the eddy currents, and consequently the rate of heat generation, will be greatest in those materials of the greatest conductivity. The relative conductivity of the various tissues of the body is about equal to their fluid content:

Muscle	72–75%
Brain	68
Fat	14–15
Skin and bone	5–16

Heating in an electromagnetic field is especially effective in vascular tissue. It is generally designated in the United States as "inductothermy."

The factors relating to coil field heating are (1) the magnitude of the coil inductance (length and shape of the coil); (2) the coil capacity (depending upon the distance between coil windings, on the magnitude of the dielectric constants of the insulating material, and on the distance from the coil to the surface of the body); and (3) the frequency of oscillation. If the frequency of the electrical energy is small compared with the natural frequency of the coil, then the coil functions inductively, by eddy current heating; if the fixed frequencies are large compared with frequency of the coil, then the coil functions capacitatively by capacitor field heating.

Microwave Heating. The newer method makes use of a radiated electromagnetic field. The energy is beamed from an antenna or radiator, and no contact is required for its transmission. This method has the limitation that the size of the antenna or radiator is inversely proportional to the frequency being transmitted. The antenna must be at least one-half wavelength long. It is obvious that an antenna 15 meters wide for radiating with a 30-meter wavelength would be impractical, whereas an antenna 1 cm wide used to radiate 2-cm waves is practical.

In human thighs, the average temperature at a depth of approximately 2 inches immediately after irradiation was 104.2° F. Gersten *et al.* found that the amount of energy absorbed by muscles after exposure to microwaves is greater than that absorbed by subcutaneous tissue or the skin; this may be due to the fact that conductivity of muscle is greater than that of fatty tissue.

Heating in Relation to Wavelength. In the developmental stage of short-wave diathermy, confusing claims were made as to difference of heating in relation to certain wavelengths, as well for so-called selective heating. In the living body, the blood flow and the rapid interchange of heat in the living tissues may render the differences in temperature negligible for all practical purposes. The variety of factors influencing tissue heating make it likewise evident that there is no optimal wavelength for heating definite tissues in the body. Wavelength in itself is not a marked factor in tissue heating, but differences in apparatus, energy delivered to the patient, and technique have important roles.

With the advent of microwave diathermy, investigations of the relative effects of microwave and short-wave heating on circulation and temperature showed some differences. However, in applying high-frequency heating from any source, one must remember that in actual practice, the uniform biological factors—the flow of blood and heat conduction to adjacent colder parts—will level off differences very considerably. As a matter of fact, clinical results with the different methods are fairly uniform as long as the current is applied within the limit of physiological toleration. It has been estimated that with short-wave diathermy in areas with normal circulation and sufficient soft tissue, uniform heating to a depth of 5 cm (2 inches) can be anticipated.

PHYSIOLOGICAL EFFECTS OF HEATING

The physiological and clinical effects of diathermy are due to the raising of the temperature of the parts under the influence of the heating currents.

The heat-regulating mechanism of the body maintains a constant temperature. When heat is applied to a part from any external source, the vasomotor mechanism responds with an effort to dissipate the excess heat. There follows an active vasodilatation of the capillaries and subsequent increase of arterial and venous circulation. Ordinarily, there is an inherent tone in the capillaries that maintains vasoconstriction. Lewis has shown that irritation of the tissues by the application of heat produces a release of vasodilator substance—histamine—which in turn results in the dilatation of the capillaries. Upon the absorption of the vasodilator substance, a greater proportion of the capillaries dilates, rather than just the few that carry blood under normal conditions; the result is a greater blood supply to the part. This local hyperemia in turn brings about an increase of the rate of removal of local tissue products. Heat increases the speed of chemical reactions occurring in the living organism. The metabolites, liberated at a great rate under the influence of heat, exert their well-known direct chemical vasodilator effect on the small-vessel bed throughout the body. This brings about two definite effects: (a) an increase in the caliber of the blood vessels and (b) an increase in the number of patent vessels; that is, in addition to the dilation of those already patent, under the influence of heat, new vascular channels are widely opened up.

While diathermy undoubtedly produces many of its effects by raising the temperature of deeper tissues, one must not lose sight of the fact that local thermal stimulation of any skin area exerts reflex reactions on deeper structures. According to physiologists, localized hyperemia of the skin is accompanied by localized hyperemia in the corresponding inner organ. The thermal stimulation of sensory receptors in the skin brings about vasodilatation through the axon reflex. Axon reflexes play an important role in the cutaneous vasodilatation observed in subjects exposed to heat. Furthermore, the sympathetic nerves are believed to contain vasodilator fibers.

When heating is applied in sufficient intensity to a large part of the body surface, *general* physiological effects arise. With a general rise in temperature of the body, the warmed blood circulating through the heat-regulating centers in the hypothalamus will bring about a discharge of impulses to increase the dissipation of heat. Consequently, a generalized vasodilatation is produced, and heat loss is increased by radiation, conduction, and convection through the skin. The pinkish skin after exposure to diathermy, hot baths, or any other source of heat is a manifestation of this generalized cutaneous vasodilatation brought about by local and central mechanisms. The heart rate may be increased by speeding up the rate of generation and propagation of impulses through the sinoatrial node.

The extent, duration, and, to a certain degree, the form of heating undoubtedly influence the aggregate of these physiological changes. However, when attempts are being made to extol the "output" of various heat generators as a major factor in bringing about effective responses, one must always be aware of the fact that only the energy that is actually absorbed by the tissues can produce an effect. It is also to be remembered that there is a time element necessary to bring about efficient heating: It appears that during the early stages of any heating for a period of about 20 minutes there is a direct relation between the energy output, the rise of temperature, and the increase of blood flow. It has also been shown that at a certain point the temperature rise in the tissues ceases after the introduction of heating energy within physiological limits; this must be due to increased removal of body heat through the increased circulation and the greater radiation from the skin.

Clinical Effects of Diathermy. The enumerated physiological effects of heating form the basis of the present-day conception of the clinical effects of diathermy as it has gradually evolved.

Effects on Circulation. LOCAL EFFECTS. The local application of diathermy results in an active arterial hyperemia that appears to be more penetrating than the hyperemia that follows external forms of heat applications. There is also an increased flow of lymph, and as a result of both hyperemia and hyperlymphia, there is an increase in the volume of the part thus affected. In glandular organs, there is a marked increase of secretion.

GENERAL EFFECTS. Diathermy applied by a method of general administration results in a dilatation of peripheral blood vessels, which appears very rapidly; this is accompanied by a rise in blood temperature, which in turn results in an increase of the pulse rate and respiration and an increase of the general body metabolism.

Effects on the Nervous System. Diathermy exerts a marked sedative effect on irritative conditions of sensory nerves (pain) and motor nerves (spasms and cramps). There is no generally accepted explanation for the pain-relieving effect. It may be that heat in some way lessens nerve sensibility, perhaps as a result of inhibition through the temperature nerves of the skin. Other investigators called attention to the fact that thermal measures exert reflex action in internal organs by stimulation of the vegetative nervous system through the nerve endings in the skin.

The sedative action on hypertonic conditions of motor nerves is generally explained by the mild heating effects. The relief of muscle cramps by heat is well known, and the effect of diathermic heat on hypertonic conditions of the unstriped muscles of the stomach and intestines is the more efficient sequel to the old-fashioned use of a hot brick to relieve colic.

8

Specific Effects Claimed for High-Frequency Energy. The possibility of effects other than heating by high-frequency currents has been a subject for speculation ever since d'Arsonval claimed specific high-frequency effects apart from those of heat. However, the only detectable effect to which therapeutic value may be ascribed is the rise in temperature that results from heat production. This rise in temperature is limited by the occurrence of burns. Consequently, effects other than thermal ones that might manifest themselves under higher intensities remain undetected. It is not possible to predict what would happen if, instead of treating tissues by means of sustained high-frequency electrical energy, tissues were subjected to intermittent radio-frequency pulses of very high intensity separated by silent periods of sufficient length to allow for the dissipation of heat.

When short-wave diathermy was first introduced, a number of specific effects were claimed for it, such as effects on capillaries and on tumors, as well as specific bactericidal action. Some observers described "athermic" effects that come about by employing only a low output of a short-wave apparatus and claimed specific influence on the autonomic and sensory nervous system. All these claims have been disproved one by one in the literature, and all the available evidence at present would indicate that besides the possibility of specific electric changes, thermal effects are the only proven biophysical effects of short-wave diathermy.

Short-Wave Diathermy vs. Microwave Diathermy. Many studies in the past have dealt with the comparative effects of short-wave and microwave diathermy. The differences in the physiological response of the body to these two forms of heating involve the extent of local heating or the degree of heating from a large amount of energy. Few studies deal with the problem. It is generally accepted that microwave, with its smaller heat output, warms the tissues locally but that the increase of local circulation rapidly dissipates the heat from the area affected. Hence, the local increase of tissue temperature is much less because of the circulatory response.

At the same time, the superficial tissues are protected against thermal damage, and there is little penetration of heat to deeper organs. In general body heating, as furnished by the more powerful short-wave apparatus, the predominant reflexes are concerned with the dissipation of heat from the body as a whole; general cardiovascular readjustments occur, and vasoconstriction occurs in such vascular beds as the renal and the splanchnic areas, which are not concerned with heat loss. This may explain the variable changes in blood flow after short-wave diathermy and the absence, in microwave diathermy, of general circulatory readjustments that often nullify the local effects.

CLINICAL USES OF DIATHERMY

The therapeutic indications for diathermy are based upon its enumerated physical and physiological effects. The heat of diathermy is generated in the tissues by the direct action of electrical energy. The placing of electrodes directly over the heated parts also prevents any appreciable cooling by evaporation.

Deep hyperemia causes an increased arterial flow with more oxygen and improved nutrition, while the greater venous flow carries away in larger degree the products of local metabolism. These effects promote disintegration of inflammatory exudates and assist in their resorption, as shown clinically by the decrease of swelling, relief of pain, and restoration of function—hence the therapeutic effectiveness of diathermy in subacute and chronic inflammatory and congestive conditions and circulatory disorders. The pain- and spasm-relieving effect of diathermy makes its use indicated in irritations of sensory and motor nerves.

Diathermy is often indicated alone; in some conditions, however, it will work to best advantage if properly combined with other physical measures, notably with those producing mechanical effects. A brief enumeration of the principal conditions in which the use of diathermy has been an effective aid in treatment is as follows:

In traumatic and inflammatory conditions of bursae, bones, and joints after the acute stage, and in painful and exuberant callus formation and fibrous ankylosis following joint injuries, diathermy or heat relieves the secondary muscle spasm and pain occurring with them.

In postoperative adhesions in extremities, diathermy may be advantageously combined with muscle exercising. Spastic conditions of the stomach, gallbladder, intestines, and pelvis of the kidney, as well as gastric neuroses, have been relieved by diathermy, though no more effectively than by other methods of heating.

In the treatment of neuritis, and in certain varieties of neuralgia or myalgia, diathermy may help to relieve pain.

In the treatment of chronic infections, many special electrodes have been designed to fit body cavities or contours. These have included rectal, vaginal, and axillary electrodes, as well as flexible electrodes cut into patterns to cover or fit the part to be treated. The effective use of antibiotics has eliminated the need to treat infected body cavities with diathermy over lengthy periods.

CONTRAINDICATIONS AND DANGERS OF DIATHERMY

Diathermy is *relatively* contraindicated in disease processes in which the usual simpler methods of superficial heat give satisfactory results. Ordinary contusions and simple myositis will readily respond to luminous heat. So, too, complicated methods recommended by some for applying diathermy to fingers and toes seem superfluous in view of the fact that such areas can be more effectively and more safely heated by radiation or hot water or paraffin baths. Superficial neuralgias and neuritis can frequently be relieved by radiant heat.

Diathermy should not be used as a panacea for all sorts of undiagnosed painful conditions. A complete diagnosis, a definite conception of the underlying pathology to be influenced, and consideration of the individual equation in each patient are essentials for its successful application.

Diathermy is *absolutely* contraindicated in three conditions: (1) In acute inflammatory processes accompanied by fever and suppuration. The pain and swelling of acutely inflamed joints in infectious arthritis are usually aggravated by diathermy, and it is almost a diagnostic evidence that the process has entered the subacute stage when diathermy can be well tolerated. In acute nondraining suppuration, such as appendicular abscess and acute pelvic infections, unwisely applied diathermy may lead to real danger by spreading the process. (2) In tendency to hemorrhage. Diathermy must not be employed in recent hemoptysis, in bleeding gastric ulcer, in large varicose veins, and in pregnancy. It is inadvisable to apply diathermy to pelvic organs during the menstrual period. (3) In malignant tumors or in case of the suspicion of such. Many authors also consider peripheral nerve injuries absolute contraindications, because the disturbed or absent skin sensitivity greatly increases the risk of burns.

The danger of burns is present in any form of thermal therapy; proper technique and the observation of all precautions are essential at all times for their prevention.

GENERAL TECHNIQUE OF DIATHERMY

General Considerations. The object of all forms of diathermy is to produce penetrating heating of the entire body or of a part of it. Effective heating will depend on the correct selection of a treatment technique, as well as on the proper dosage and duration of the treatment.

The selection of the method of treatment and particular technique—electric or electromagnetic field or direct conduction heating—will depend on the available apparatus and on the condition to be treated in the individual patient. Generally speaking, all forms of diathermy when applied intelligently will result in satisfactory deep tissue heating. Certain techniques are, however, preferable because of convenience or safety for certain locations and certain pathological conditions.

Regulation of Dosage. Medical diathermy must be a pleasant procedure at all times and must never cause pain during treatment or damage to the tissues. As a general rule, the strength of current should be no more, at any time, than that which feels comfortable to the individual patient. We do not have any practical device for the exact measurement of the heat attained in the interior of the body. The meter in short-wave apparatus serves only as an indicator that electrical energy is passing; it does not register the amount of energy passing through the patient. "Dosimeters" have been constructed for short-wave apparatus to measure the power absorption by the patient, but they have not stood the test of general clinical use.

The *heat sensation* of the patient is the supreme guide of dosage in all diathermy treatments. Hence the physician must be certain at all times that the patient perceives heat normally, and in doubtful cases, testing with test tubes filled with hot and cold water should be done. A definite excess amount of current will manifest itself by an unpleasant burning sensation in the skin or a feeling of pressure in the subcutaneous tissues. Patients complain of the latter, especially when too much current is crowded into a narrow area, such as the wrist or ankle, in longitudinal (cuff) application.

Short-wave diathermy should produce a smooth, "velvety" sensation of heat. Four grades of heat sensation in short-wave treatments have been established by several clinicians: (1) threshold value (glowlike sensation); (2) distinct feeling of agreeable warmth; (3) intensive heat; (4) unbearable heat. For very mild dosage, as in acutely painful conditions, one should stay within the glowlike sensation, while in chronic cases, the sensation should be just this side of intensive heat.

A rapid rise of heating by fairly strong amounts of energy is not desirable in deep heating. In treating internal organs, especially the thoracic, abdominal, and pelvic organs, a moderate amount of current and comparatively long treatment produces better effects. Regarding short-wave diathermy, the temperature in the deep tissue rises in a straight line until near the end of the 20-minute treatment period. After treatment, the final temperature is actually much lower. This may be also explained by the rapid dissipation of heat by the increased blood circulation. Weaker currents to the limbs are indicated, as a general rule, in acute painful conditions, such as in acute neuritis and recent cases of traumatism and also in chronic arthritis with marked trophic changes. In treatment of acute inflammatory conditions by short-wave diathermy, best results have been achieved with 10-minute applications of low intensity.

Duration and Frequency of Treatment. It is evident that it takes a certain amount of time for the temperature of the part treated to reach the desired level; then, through automatic heat regulation, a condition of equilibrium will ensue so that a fairly constant temperature is maintained. It is also evident that superficial parts can be heated in less time than deepseated structures; therefore, longer treatments are indicated for inner organs.

Clinical experience has established that *20 minutes* is the minimum time required for an efficient diathermy treatment in limbs or superficial parts of the body. In treatment of internal organs, about one-half hour is advisable. Excessively long treatments may cause too intensive a heat effect and thereby exhaust the patient, especially if he is aged.

Acute and very painful conditions or recent injuries in which the early return of function is essential, as a rule, require daily treatment. With improvement of such conditions, this repetition can be reduced. For the average patient suffering from some chronic ailment, treatment on alternate days usually suffices and may even be administered less often, depending upon the progress noted.

As a general rule, therapeutic applications of heat are most effective when repeated three or four times a day. This is not practical in hospital or office practice. For this reason, simple methods of heating that may be safely used in the home according to specific instructions are most useful. For a few special conditions, diathermy may be effective when applied daily or on alternate days. This is true in the case of bursitis of the shoulder and hip regions and in some cases of low back strain.

TECHNIQUE OF SHORT-WAVE DIATHERMY

Electrodes. Each of the forms of short-wave diathermy application involves the use of different types of electrodes:

Electric or condenser field heating	Flexible condenser pads, air-spaced plates, single and double cuffs
Electromagnetic field heating	Inductance cable wound around part or placed upon body in form of a loop, pancake coil, or treatment drum

Electric or Condenser Field Heating. Electric field heating consists of applying two spaced metal electrodes—condenser pads and cuffs or air-spaced electrodes—on either opposite surfaces or the same body surface to heat the interposed part. (See Fig. 16–1 and Fig. 16–7.)

Condenser pads are held in place by elastic bandaging or perforated rubber bands or by some other suitable means, such as sandbags or by the patient resting on them. The advantage of pads is their pliability, which allows bending or shaping them to conform with the surface to be treated. The rubber insulation of imperfectly jointed or pressed pads may puncture, with subsequent danger of arcing and burns through the exposed part of the metal. For this reason, and to avoid overheating the skin, the pads should never be placed directly over the skin; a dry towel or some other dry insulating material such as perforated felt, of at least $1/4$-inch thickness, should be interposed. In applying the pads, care must be taken that their cable connection nowhere directly touches the patient's skin.

Accumulation of moisture due to perspiration under the electrodes leads to a concentration of electrical energy near the skin and the possibility of superficial burns. Hence, it is a general rule to place, in addition

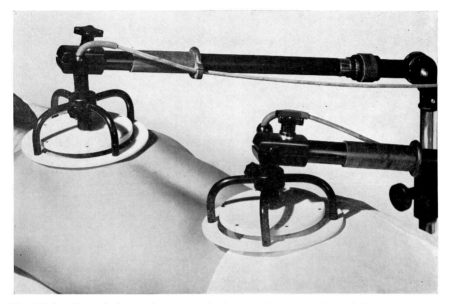

Fig. 16–1. Spaced plates, short-wave diathermy. (Courtesy of Burdick Corporation.)

to suitable spacing, moisture-absorbing material between the electrodes and the skin. If turkish towels are used for spacing, this is not necessary; in all other cases, linen or paper towels, thin blotting paper, or tissue paper should be employed. Felt pads used for spacing should always be free from moisture.

Double cuffs consist of a pair of long, narrow condenser pads that are applied along a limb at suitable distance from each other. They should be so placed that they include only the part to be heated, and the skin-electrode distance under both cuffs should be equal. It makes no difference if part of one cuff overlaps the other.

Air-spaced condenser plates consist of circular metal plates or discs covered with insulating material. The plates are mounted on adjustable treatment arms and are self-retaining in any desired position (Fig. 16–1). This is especially convenient over the thighs and shoulders.

The correct spacing of these various forms of electrodes is quite a problem. Generally speaking, the thicker the part of the body to be treated, the greater should be the skin-electrode distance and the greater should be the size of the electrodes. It is important to follow the instructions given by the manufacturers for the correct spacing in relation to the power ouput of their apparatus. Figure 16–2 diagrammatically shows the influence of spacing on the underlying tissues. Under certain conditions, it may be desirable to produce more surface heating on one side and more depth effect on the other; this can be done by using less spacing on one side and more on the other.

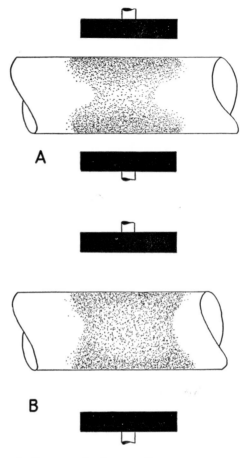

Fig. 16–2.   Schematic diagram of influence of spacing on extent of depth effect. A, close spacing, more superficial heating; B, wider spacing, more depth heating.

Electromagnetic or Coil Field Heating. Coil field heating or inducto-thermy serves for heating an entire extremity or part of it. To treat an entire limb or a joint, two to four thicknesses of turkish toweling should be placed between the cable and the skin. There should be two to four turns of the cable wound round the part to be treated, depending on its size; these turns should be spaced 1 inch or more apart; convenient wooden "spacers" serve for this purpose. In all inductance cable treatments, the ends of the cable leading to the apparatus should be of equal length and should be separated by at least the distance of the outlets on the apparatus (Fig. 16–3).

Instead of winding an inductance cable around a limb, it can be applied in the form of a pancake or held in a so-called treatment drum (Fig. 16–4). In this form, it can be applied on any part of the body, held at a

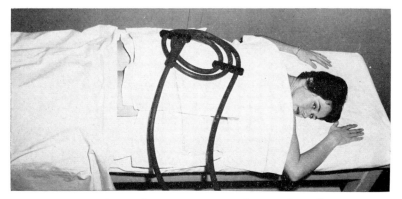

Fig. 16–3.   Short-wave treatment by pancake coil.

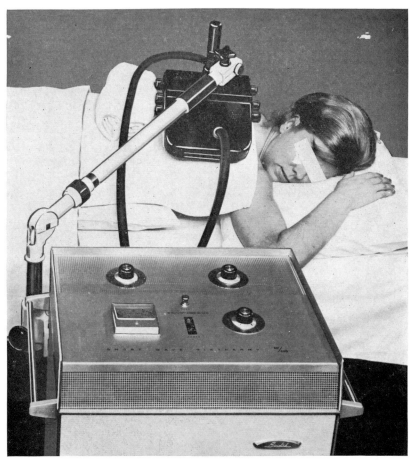

Fig. 16–4.   Hinged-drum application to upper back.
(Courtesy of Burdick Corporation.)

proper distance by interposition of spacing by towels or by air. The turns of the pancake coil should be about 1 inch apart. The advantage of this type of electrode is its convenience of application to anatomical location.

TECHNIQUE OF MICROWAVE DIATHERMY

When microwave diathermy was first introduced, there were four different directors, which were applied at varying distances from the body for the production of a specific heating pattern. The size and configuration of each pattern was dependent on two functions: (1) the spacing between director and patient and (2) the shape of the reflector. More recently, a large corner-type E director has been developed (Fig. 16–5), and this is becoming the standard director, although the A and B directors are optional when buying a microwave unit.

Directors A and B are made in the form of hemispheres of 4 inches and 6 inches in diameter, respectively. These directors produce circular patterns with the maximum heating in the periphery. This feature serves to equalize skin temperatures when treating irregular surfaces. Director E is a corner reflector type, and it produces an ovate pattern with maximum heating in the center. This provides more uniform heating over relatively smooth or concave body areas. The minimum spacing with any director is 1 inch, the maximum varying from 2 inches in the case of the

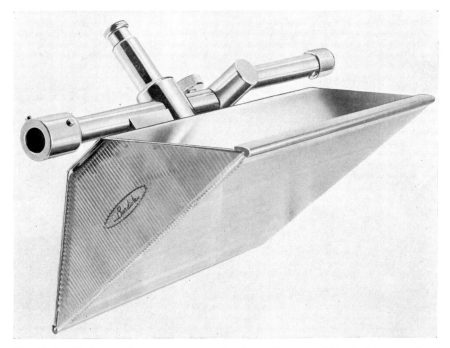

Fig. 16–5. E director for microwave application. (Courtesy of Burdick Corporation.)

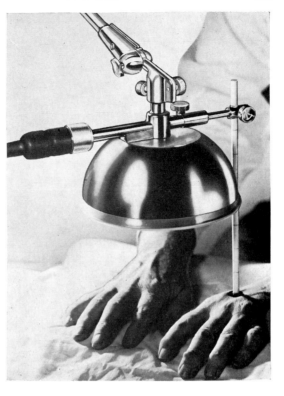

Fig. 16–6. Microwave spacer gauge with B director. (Courtesy of Burdick Corporation.)

A director to 6 inches in the case of the E director. At close spacings, the pattern of heating is smaller. With increased spacing, the area covered increases.

As can readily be seen, the directors for microwave application are applied at a fairly close approximation. A spacer gauge allows the operator to set the desired spacing (Fig. 16–6).

The power ouput must be adjusted to accommodate the various areas. As a general rule, when treating small areas using close spacing, the power required is very low. As the area treated increases, the space increases, and greater power is necessary. The power output meter itself has been calibrated in percentage of power rather than in milliamperes, with the greatest available power being marked 100 per cent. Depending on the director employed and the spacing required, the power output will vary from 15–20 per cent for a small area to 100 per cent for a large area. (See Table 16–1.)

As in all heat treatments, the determination of power output and length of treatments is a matter for judgment and experience. The power output level should always be within the comfortable surface tolerance of the patient. The length of treatment should be 15 to 20 minutes.

In applying microwave diathermy, one should see that the surfaces treated are dry, and no toweling should be placed over the skin. Accumu-

Table 16–1. Relation of Director Spacing to Power Output

Spacing (in.) Director E	Meter Reading (%)
1	20–40
2	40–60
3	60–80
4	80–90
5–6	90–100
Director B (6-in. hemisphere)	
2	40–50
3	60–80
4	100

lated moisture can be wiped off from time to time. The directors should not be used without their protective coverings; otherwise, accidental contact with the tips of the radiators and immediate burns may occur. The directors should never be placed with the open side against the metal surface of a table when the power is on, as this will cause irreparable damage to the magnetron tube. The microwave unit should be properly grounded at all times; this will protect the operator from possible injury. *Watches should be kept away from the high-frequency electric fields because of the danger of magnetizing.*

Microwave heating cannot be used at present for orifice heating; neither can it be used for the treatment of large surfaces or of entire limbs. It is well suited for efficient heating of circumscribed areas, and because of its more uniform absorption rate as compared to the two other forms of diathermic heating, it may avoid overheating of superficially located tissues.

Special care is advised when treating the region of the head, especially the eyes. Investigations by Worden *et al.* showed that the temperature tolerated by normal tissue cannot be regarded as a safe range of tolerance for ischemic tissues. Others have found that cataractous lenticular opacities are produced in rabbit eye 2 to 40 days after a series of exposures of a smaller magnitude, as well after a single direct exposure. It was also found that bony prominences are potential sites for formation of blebs, undoubtedly due to current concentration.

REGIONAL TECHNIQUE OF DIATHERMY

The general principles of application of short-wave and microwave diathermy to various regions and organs are in many respects similar. They allow quite a variety of application and flexibility of technique in many locations and conditions. The ease with which microwave is applied makes it a useful method of heating individual joints of both the upper and lower extremities.

Neck. The cervical spine may be treated with condenser pads either anteroposteriorly (a narrower pad over the cervical spine, a dispersive

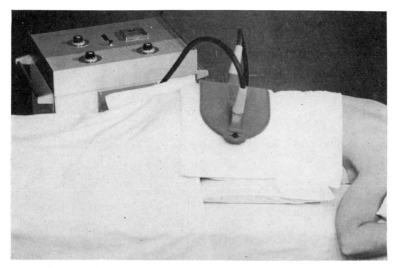

Fig. 16–7. Treatment of lower back with condenser pads.
(Courtesy of Burdick Corporation.)

pad over the upper anterior chest) or laterally (two equal-sized pads on each side of the neck). Spaced plates may also be applied. All structures of the neck may be treated by several turns of an inductance cable, wrapped around several thicknesses of turkish toweling. Finally, a few turns of the pancake coil may be placed over the cervical spine with toweling interposed. Microwave diathermy can be simply focused by an applicator.

Dorsal and Lumbar Spine. The dorsal and lumbar spine may be treated with a pancake coil with the patient lying prone (Fig. 16–3). Condenser pads may also be used for these areas (Fig. 16–7). Microwave diathermy allows easy application in either sitting or abdominal recumbent position.

Coccyx. Treatment is similar to low back technique using pancake coil or drum. An alternative method is to place the drum under a wooden chair upon which the patient sits. This technique has been used in treating the prostate and perineal areas. Another method is to have the patient sit on a pancake coil padded with several layers of turkish toweling.

Shoulder and Upper Limb. The irregular contour of the shoulder presents quite a task for efficient and comfortable application of diathermy. As a general rule, in order to relax all structures, the patient should be reclining on a treatment couch with the arm abducted and propped up by supporting pillows. Short-wave treatment may be given by a pancake coil or loop placed over several layers of toweling or by spaced plates held anteroposteriorly by treatment arms. For treatment of both shoulders, a spaced plate may be placed over each shoulder. Microwave diathermy is especially convenient for one shoulder, an elbow, or hand (Fig. 16–6).

Elbow. Treatment may be rendered by an inductance cable wrapped around a flexible drum. When the elbow cannot be fully extended, the cuff method of heating should not be applied, since it will lead to undue current concentration on the flexor surface of the joint.

Wrist and Hand. The inductance cable method is quite effective, either in the form of a loop wound around the parts or with the hand placed over a pancake coil. The hand also can be treated by being placed between two large flexible condenser pads. Fingers can be heated jointly or singly by being placed in contact with one condenser pad, while the other pad is placed behind the arm, the elbow being held in flexion.

For the treatment of the entire upper or lower limb, either an inductance cable or flexible drum can be employed.

Hip and Thigh. The pancake coil technique can be employed by placing a few turns of the inductance cable directly over the region to be treated. The flexible drum is equally effective.

Knee. The knee should always be treated with the patient on a table or couch. The inductance cable is quite convenient; several turns should be wound around the knee. The same technique can be employed for treating both knees simultaneously. The flexible drum is also applicable (Fig. 16–8).

Ankle and Foot. The ankle can be treated by an inductance cable wound around it (Fig. 16–9). It may be also treated by a condenser pad under the heel and foot and a circular cuff placed around the middle of the leg. The foot can be treated by similar technique. Both feet and legs can be warmed up by pad electrodes placed under the sole of each foot. It is important that both electrodes be kept at suitable distance from the floor to avoid loss of energy by grounding.

Sciatic Nerve. Short-wave diathermy may be applied by an inductance cable wound around the lower limb, by two condenser pads, or by

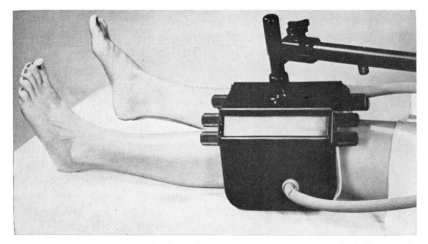

Fig. 16–8.   Treatment of knee by hinged electrode. (Courtesy of Burdick Corporation.)

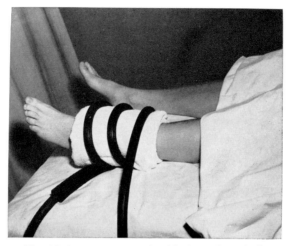

Fig. 16–9.   Treatment of ankle by coil method.

two air-spaced plates, one placed over the lumbar or gluteal region, the other on the posterior aspect of the thigh just above the knee. After 20 minutes of treatment, this electrode is moved to the middle of the calf, and 20 minutes more treatment may be applied.

Safety Rules in All Diathermy Treatments. In addition to the general rules for electric treatment, the following special rules are to be observed in applying all diathermy treatments:

1. Before applying electrodes, carefully inspect the parts to be treated to make sure that the continuity of the skin is nowhere broken and that the heat sensation of the patient is normal. In case of scar tissue, peripheral nerve injuries, or hysterical anesthesia, be extremely careful in the application of diathermy.

2. Before turning on the current from the main inlet, inform the patient that the sensation to be expected is that of mild heat. Instruct the patient to report any uncomfortable sensation, pricking, or burning at once.

3. After starting the current through the main switch, open up the current regulator gradually. In some short-wave apparatus, one control serves to regulate the current; in others, a separate tuning control must be set first.

4. Do not try to push the current up to the maximum amount of toleration during the first few treatments. Patients often are burned in their endeavor to show how much current they can stand. Remember the principle that a moderate amount of heat applied for a longer period is more effective than pushing up to the limit of tolerance for a shorter period.

5. If at any time during the treatment the patient complains of an uncomfortable sensation anywhere, turn off the controls, shutting off the main current inlet in case of emergency, and, if necessary, take off, inspect, and reapply the electrodes. When inspecting or adjusting elec-

trodes, be sure that the current is turned off and increased gradually again after such a procedure.

6. Do not leave the patient alone during treatment unless you have arranged that by the simple pulling of a cord or the turning of a switch, the patient himself can turn off the current at any time. Watch the milliammeter during the entire treatment for an even flow of the current.

7. At the end of the treatment, turn off the controls in the reverse order to which they have been turned on. This will leave all the switches and controls in safe position to start the next treatment. Take off the electrodes carefully and inspect the site of application each time.

8. Let the patient rest after treatment long enough to make sure that the skin has fully cooled off, especially in inclement weather.

Correct application of diathermy in various conditions can be learned only through ample clinical instruction. It is not fair to reputable manufacturers to expect their salesmen to be instructors in technique.

Special Precautions with Short-Wave Diathermy. In applying short-wave treatment, metallic objects, such as hairpins, safety pins, buttons, keys, knives, watches, and buckles should be removed from the field of treatment because they lead to a concentration of electrical energy and the possibility of arcing and burns. Metallic chairs or tables, radiators, water pipes, electric fixtures, or other grounded metal should not be within possible contact with the patient; nor should conducting cables make contact with such objects. Hence it is preferable to use treatment tables and chairs without metallic parts and to use mattresses without metal innersprings.

Special care must be taken that no cables leading to the apparatus cut across each other or get too close to each other, because this may lead to overheating of their insulation and possible fire.

Like all other electrical treatments, short-wave diathermy should be applied to the unclothed body only. Application of electrodes over the clothed parts breeds carelessness in observance of the elementary rule of close inspection of the parts before and after treatment; also, the varying thickness of clothing may interfere with correct spacing of the electrodes. Hidden metal objects as well as unsuspected moisture in the clothing are also potential causes for burns.

Embedded Metals. Operative implantation of metals in the body tissues, as increasingly practiced in recent years, has brought up the problem of the postoperative use of diathermy in these cases, and for a while the dictum prevailed that diathermy cannot be used. Studies by Etter *et al.* disclosed, however, that on histological examination, tissues contiguous to metals showed no evidence of destructive effects from diathermy under ordinary treatment conditions. To a certain extent, this appears to agree with earlier findings on equalization of heat in the deeper tissues. Another study by Lion corroborated the fact that when metals are embedded deep in the tissues, the field concentration is of little practical significance; however, overheating of tissues may still occur around large metallic parts located on or near the surface. The same findings were made with microwave heating. Hence it may be safely stated that when surgical metals are situated in the deep tissues and no evidence of impaired circulation is noted, there is no danger of undue overheating with short-wave and microwave diathermy when standard clinical intensities are applied with careful technique.

ADDITIONAL READING

Downey, J. A., Darling, R. C., and Miller, J. M.: The effect of heat, cold, and exercise on the peripheral circulation. Arch. Phys. Med. Rehab., 49:308, 1969.

Etter, H. S., Pudenz, R. H., and Gersh, I.: The effect of diathermy on tissues contiguous to implanted surgical metals. Arch. Phys. Med. Rehab., 28:333, 1947.

Gersten, J. W., Wakim, K. G., Herrick, J. F., and Krusen, F. H.: The effect of microwave diathermy on peripheral circulation and on tissue temperatures in man. Arch. Phys. Med. Rehab., 30:7, 1949.

Lehmann, J. F.: Diathermy, pp. 244–327. In F. H. Krusen, F. J. Kottke, and P. M. Ellwood, Jr. (ed.), Handbook of Physical Medicine and Rehabilitation. W. B. Saunders Co., Philadelphia, 1965.

Lehmann, J. F., McMillian, J. A., Brunner, G. D., and Blumberg, J. B.: Comparative study of the efficiency of shortwave, microwave, and ultrasonic diathermy in heating the hip joint. Arch. Phys. Med. Rehab., 40:510, 1959.

Lewis, T.: The Blood Vessels of the Human Skin and Their Responses. Shaw and Sons, London, 1927.

Lion, K. S.: The effect of the presence of metals in tissues subjected to diathermy treatment. Arch. Phys. Med. Rehab., 28:345, 1947.

Moor, F. B.: Microwave diathermy, pp. 310–320. In S. Licht (ed.), Therapeutic Heat and Cold. 2nd ed. Waverly Press, Baltimore, 1965.

Richardson, A. W., Duane, T. D., and Hines, H. M.: Experimental lenticular opacities produced by microwave irradiation. Arch. Phys. Med. Rehab., 29:765, 1948.

Scott, B. O.: Short wave diathermy, pp. 279– 309. In S. Licht (ed.), Therapeutic Heat and Cold. 2nd ed. Waverly Press, Baltimore, 1965.

Worden, R. E., Herrick, J. F., Wakim, K. G., and Krusen, F. H.: The heating effects of microwave diathermy with and without ischemia. Arch. Phys. Med. Rehab., 29:751, 1948.

PART VII

Ultrasound

Chapter 17

ULTRASOUND

History. The biological effects of ultrasound were first noted by Langevin when he observed that small fish were killed when they swam into a beam of ultrasonic waves. It was about 1917 when he envisioned practical applications of this type of energy and made ultrasound more than theoretical research. Robert Williams Wood, an American physicist, worked with Langevin, and in 1927 he and Loomis published results of biological interest. In the following years, reports on the biological effects of ultrasound appeared in numerous publications. It was probably Horvath's studies in 1944 that gave ultrasound its greatest impetus in medicine. His reports were of the successful treatment by ultrasound of sarcomatous disease in human skin as well as other types of superficial malignant growths. The use of ultrasound in medicine grew rapidly in Europe, particularly in Germany, but its adoption in this country was slower and was accompanied by more skepticism. In 1952, the Council on Physical Medicine and Rehabilitation presented its first report on the status of ultrasonic energy, indicating that this physical agent had come of age in the United States. Medical literature is now filled with clinical reports of its effectiveness, and more knowledge of its biological effects comes from the laboratories of basic science daily. Echograms of the heart, aorta, eye, and brain are now used in the diagnosis of conditions of displacement or enlargement of these organs.

Physics. Although ultrasonic energy is a mechanical vibration identical to that of sound but of higher frequency, it is produced from electrical energy that is transformed into mechanical energy. Because its source is a high-frequency current, it is included in this manual of electrotherapy.

The first step in producing ultrasound energy is generation of a high-frequency alternating current similar to the usual diathermy generator. In clinical practice today, frequencies vary between 30,000 and 1 million cycles per second. As the upper limit of detection of sound by human ears is set at about 20,000 cycles per second, the term ultrasound is applied to these inaudible high-frequency vibrations. This should not be confused with supersonics, which refers to *speeds* greater than the velocity of sound. The electrical energy is most commonly converted into

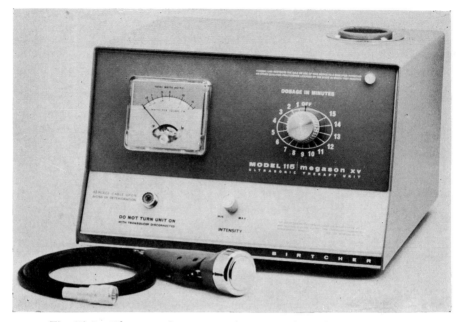

Fig. 17-1.   Ultrasonic therapy unit. (Courtesy of Birtcher Corporation.)

mechanical vibrations by means of a piezoelectric crystal. One of the most satisfactory and most commonly used crystals is barium titanate ($BaTiO_3$). Other crystals used are quartz (SiO_2) and lithium sulfate ($LiSO_4$). Quartz is the most stable material, but it requires a high voltage and, consequently, a large-diameter coaxial cable. The high-frequency field is impressed upon the crystal, usually in the neighborhood of 1 million times per second. Since quartz has high impedance, it requires high voltage. Barium titanate, on the other hand, requires very little voltage. This is a ceramic material and not a natural crystal. Of medium impedance is lithium sulfate. It is a perfect crystal but is grown from a "seed" and does not appear naturally.

At an output of 3 watts per square centimeter, quartz may require approximately 2000 volts; barium, 100; and lithium, 500. At the same time, the amperage changes inversely, as the product of volts and amperes must be constant (watts = volts × amperes).

Construction of Crystal. The crystal is cemented to the metal face of the transducer, making a ground connection. Against the back of the crystal is a pillbox-shaped area filled with air; air is a very good reflector of ultrasonic waves, whereas sound is generally carried better through solids and liquids. The air, accordingly, reflects the sound to the using end of the transducer. This plate must be tuned to the oscillation of the crystal, which is related to the sound wavelength. It is, of course, important that there be a good coupling between the transducer and the body surface to which it is applied. Poor coupling causes surface burning, which is different from the deep pain from deep penetration of energy and the production of heat.

It is of interest to point out some of the differences between electromagnetic waves and sound waves. The electromagnetic waves travel at a velocity of 3×10^8 meters per second, whereas ultrasonic waves in air travel around 330 meters per second. The velocity of sound at room temperature in fluid is about 1,450 meters per second.

Ultrasound energy is measured in watts. The total wattage is that given off by the total surface of the crystal, or the metal applicator covering it. For instance, if the total wattage is 10 and the area is 5 square centimeters, the sound head is delivering 2 watts per square centimeter average power. We use the term watts per square centimeter in the prescription for ultrasound and in determining the proper dial setting on the generator. Most machines have a calibrated meter from which may be read either the total wattage (Fig. 17–1) or watts per square centimeter, or both. These clinical generators deliver power with a total wattage of not more than 15, or 3 watts per square centimeter. In clinical practice, power levels rarely exceed 2 watts per square centimeter.

Physiological Effects. Because of the penetrating heat effects of ultrasound, it is often called diathermy. Ultrasonic diathermy, however, has some unique effects. It causes increased heating at interfaces such as junctions between different tissues such as bone and muscle. In animal studies, cavitation has been seen to occur in tissues with excessive dosage. This does not occur with dosage used clinically. There also seems to be selective heating of bones, joints, tendons, and nerves. High-dosage, focused ultrasound may be used to destroy peripheral neuromas and to produce brain lesions. Surgically implanted metal used in treatment of fractures or in arthroplasties has acoustical impedance much greater than surrounding soft tissues. This can lead to reflection and focusing of standing waves. Selective heating, however, is dependent on such factors as rate of dissipation of heat through conduction and convection and the specific heats of the metal and tissues. Further studies are needed before definite clinical conclusions can be drawn, although at dosage levels normally used, no undue heating has been reported. The destructive effect of ultrasound on tumor cells has been proven, but this is not considered a proper method of treatment at the present time because the disease cannot be eradicated by this method since islets of tumor will still remain.

Comparative Heating with Short-Wave, Microwave, and Ultrasonic Diathermy. Conversion of electromagnetic radiations such as the short-wave and microwave diathermy and of acoustical radiation (ultrasound) results in deeper heating in tissues than conductive heating. Experimental studies have shown that bones and joints covered by relatively little soft tissue may be heated by diathermy and ultrasound diathermy.

Technique of Application. The general rules of technique in applying diathermy can be used for ultrasound diathermy. The patient must be comfortably positioned, depending on the area of the body to be treated, and the skin should be examined before the treatment, tested for presence of sensation, and inspected after the treatment. Ultrasound is often followed by other physical therapeutic procedures.

Ultrasound generators require a short period of warming up before they are ready to be used. There is usually a dial for tuning the sound head with the oscillating circuit; this is done until a maximum meter reading is obtained. The output dial is then set so that the desired reading is obtained, usually in a range between 1 and 2 watts per square centimeter. Most generators have a built-in timing device that automatically shuts off the machine at the end of the treatment.

Direct Oil Coupling.   The most common method of transmitting ultrasound from the sound head to the skin and underlying tissues is by means of a coupling with mineral oil or similar material (Fig. 17–2). It is essential that there be no air gaps between the sound head and the underlying skin, so an ample amount of oil must be used at all times. Since some excess oil is apt to run off, it is customary to protect the patient by draping him with bath towels.

During the treatment, the sound head is slowly moved back and forth either in a rotary or transverse method in order to reduce the concentration of energy at any one point. The direct pressure applied through the sound head to the skin is not heavy but should be firm enough to maintain a good oil coupling. The length of treatment will vary in the individual case and is up to the physician. Average duration varies between 5 and 10 minutes. Some manufacturers have produced pulsating waves that reduce the average wattage output, thus lessening the necessity for the movement of the sound head during therapy.

Underwater Coupling.   The sound heads of the generators are so constructed that they may be placed under water, sometimes with the help of a handle. The advantage of this technique is that bony prominences or concave surfaces that could not be efficiently coupled by means of oil

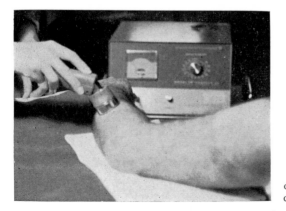

Fig. 17–2.   Ultrasonic application to the elbow with oil coupling.

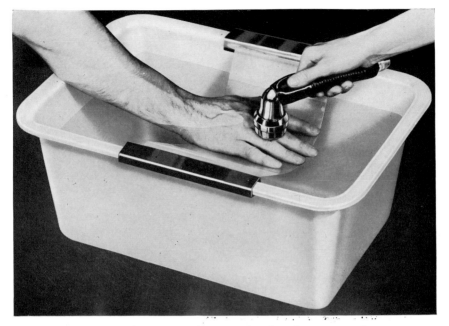

Fig. 17–3. Ultrasonic application to hand, underwater coupling.
(Courtesy of Birtcher Corporation.)

can be treated using the coupling medium of water in a bath, such as a whirlpool bath or any suitably sized container. This method of application is also used where the surface to be treated is particularly sensitive. For example, in treating a painful neuroma that will not tolerate direct pressure, the area may be immersed in water and the sound head held about 1 to 1½ inches from the area without producing painful sensations. The underwater method is particularly useful in treating hands, feet, and elbows (Fig. 17–3).

The frequency of treatment is always determined individually. To begin with, treatments may be given daily and then reduced in frequency when desired effects are noted. It is often observed that 1 to 3 hours after treatment there may be an increase in discomfort followed later by diminished pain and an overall beneficial effect. Many observers have also felt that it requires as many as three to six treatments before the beneficial effects become apparent.

A more recent technique of giving ultrasound is called "diasonic." This consists essentially of a sound applicator 3 inches in diameter (Fig. 17–4). This applicator is held in the desired position against the skin of the back, hand, etc., with a little force so that, with application of mineral oil, a firm coupling is secured. The therapist, having set the patient up in a comfortable position for the area to be treated, simply adds the mineral oil and turns the dials for the prescribed dosage in watts per square

9

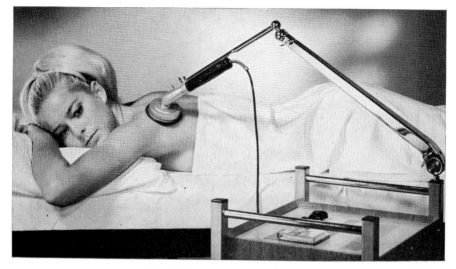

Fig. 17–4.   Diasonic applicator.

centimeters. Four to 6 watts is an average dosage level, for example, in the case of calcific bursitis.

The time of treatment is maintained by a built-in timing device controlled by the therapist or physician. This is usually set for 10 or 15 minutes. The additional application of local heat in the form of hot pack or infrared is optional and dependent on the physician's orders. The same is true for massage and exercises to increase range of motion.

This method of applying ultrasound is easier than conventional methods using rotary or stroking motions.

Another recent method of ultrasound application is the combination of electrical stimulation with ultrasound in one unit.

Clinical Applications.   Ultrasound therapy, as well as microwave and short-wave diathermy, is generally used with other forms of physical procedures in the treatment of various conditions involving muscles, bones, and joints.   Hydrotherapy and therapeutic exercises may be combined with ultrasound to advantage.   Those conditions for which ultrasound seems to have a specific therapeutic advantage over other forms of therapy will be discussed.

Bursitis or Tendinitis of the Shoulder.   Many cases of acute pain in the shoulder diagnosed as bursitis or tendinitis with or without calcium deposits may respond to daily or alternate-day applications of ultrasound to the shoulder region (Fig. 17–5). If relief is not obtained in 3 or 4 treatments, it is usually best to stop ultrasound and change the method of treatment to the use of ice packs, rest, and aspirin. Frequently, injections of novocain with or without hydrocortone are useful. Ultrasound has not been particularly effective in the chronic cases of frozen shoulder with severe

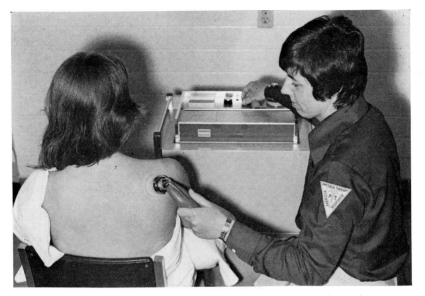

Fig. 17–5. Ultrasonic treatment of the shoulder with oil coupling.

limitation of motion. For these cases, simpler forms of heat, such as hot packs, and, particularly, carefully graduated exercises are employed.

Bursitis in the Hip Region. Diagnosis is made clinically by point tenderness in the region of the bursa over the trochanter of the femur and in the gluteal muscle insertions and is occasionally confirmed by roentgenographic evidence of calcium deposits. A certain percentage of patients respond to ultrasound therapy, much as do certain shoulder cases. The same technique of application is used.

Cervical Strain. Cases of ligamentous strain in the cervical region are frequent; they are called whiplash injuries if they occur after automobile accidents. Clinical findings include spasm of the cervical muscles, sometimes unilateral, producing a certain degree of torticollis; there may also be some signs of radicular involvement with paresthesias, pain, and occasionally numbness extending down the arm and into the hand. The majority of cases improve with simple measures, including, applications of heat, rest, and protection with a collar. Occasionally, patients derive benefit from the use of gentle head traction. Recovery may be slow, but it is frequently hastened by application of ultrasound to the cervical muscles in combination with the other methods mentioned. The exact benefit of ultrasound is frequently difficult to evaluate objectively in chronic conditions because of the common occurrence of emotional lability.

Low Back Strain. Ultrasound treatment (Fig. 17–6) may be combined with rest, hydrotherapy, and the use of crutches and therapeutic exercises as tolerated. When there are signs of nerve root irritation with sciatica

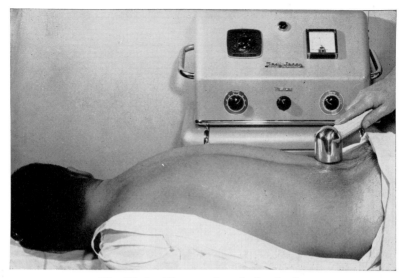

Fig. 17–6. Ultrasound applied to back.

present, benefit may occasionally be seen from ultrasound application paravertebrally in the region of the posterior roots, combined with application to the sciatic nerve as it emerges from the sciatic notch. Daily treatments for one week may be tried and continued less frequently thereafter if there is some improvement.

Neuromas. Ultrasound has a more or less specific beneficial effect on neuromas such as are seen in relation to digital nerve injuries of the hands and feet and also on stump neuromas after limb amputation. Daily applications are used with direct oil coupling for 6 to 8 minutes with 1.5 to 2 watts per cm^2 for six treatments followed by less frequent application as improvement occurs. In post-thoracotomy patients, one also occasionally finds a syndrome of thoracic neuromas that may be treated similarly, often with good results. In the case of extremely painful hypersensitive neuromas, application through underwater coupling may be necessary in the beginning.

Herpes Zoster Neuralgia. Chronic segmental pain is seen all too frequently following herpes zoster. About 50 per cent of the cases derive benefit from ultrasound application using techniques described for neuromas.

Scar Tissue. Ultrasound is thought to have a beneficial effect in loosening scar tissue, even in the treatment of Dupuytren's contracture. A course of 6 to 10 treatments may be tried.

Athletic Injuries. Frequent reports from trainers and occasionally from surgeons treating athletic injuries have indicated beneficial effects from ultrasound applications. Ultrasound has been used for the usual football injuries involving the ankles, knees, and shoulders, beginning treatment 48 to 72 hours after the acute injury. Diagnosis was usually contusions and ligamentous strain, without fracture or more serious injury. These were all college students eager to get back into the game as soon as possible, and they seemed to respond with some relief of pain to daily applications for about 1 week. These treatments were frequently combined with whirlpool baths, always preceded by pressure bandaging in the acute state and by support later. Exercises were added when judged safe by the attending surgeon. Results of studies of similar injuries over the years indicated that ultrasound may have relieved pain in the early stages but that the total time required for recovery was not substantially shortened by the addition of ultrasound to the therapeutic agents commonly used.

Ulcers. Chronic varicose ulcers of the limbs have been reported to respond to local application of ultrasound. As venous disease may also be accompanied by obstructive arterial disease, ultrasound should be used with caution, if at all. Decubitus ulcers have been reported to respond to ultrasound treatments. It is not clear from the reports available whether the better results were due to the ultrasound or to the better nursing care in the patients receiving such therapy.

Contraindications. Because of the possibility of injuring nervous tissue, ultrasound should not be applied in or about the brain, spinal cord, eye, ear, heart, reproductive organs, epiphyses of growing bones or the large autonomic structures, such as the celiac, mesenteric, and stellate ganglions. Ultrasound is also contraindicated in areas of the body where there is impaired circulation, as from occlusive vascular disease, or where sensation is impaired. Ultrasound should not be applied in acute infections or to malignant lesions.

ADDITIONAL READING

Gersten, J. W.: Effect of metallic objects on temperature rises produced in tissue by ultrasound. Am. J. Phys. Med., 37:75, 1958.

Howry, D. H.: A brief atlas of diagnostic ultrasonic radiologic results. Radiol. Clin. N. Amer., 3:433, 1965.

Lehmann, J. F.: Ultrasound therapy, pp. 321–386. In S. Licht (ed.), *Therapeutic Heat and Cold.* 2nd ed. Waverly Press, Baltimore, 1965.

Lehmann, J. F., DeLateur, B. J., Warren, C. G., and Stonebridge, J. B.: Heating of joint structures by ultrasound. Arch. Phys. Med. Rehab., 49:29, 1968.

Vaughen, J. L., and Bender, L. F.: Effects of ultrasound on growing bone. Arch. Phys. Med. Rehab., 40:158, 1959.

GLOSSARY

Actinic. Pertaining to actinism. Capable of producing chemical changes as applied to radiant energy. Usually applied to radiant energy having this property.

Actinotherapy. Treatment of disease by rays of light, especially actinic or chemical light.

Action spectrum. A plotted curve relating the wavelength of light and its effectiveness in producing a given photobiologic response.

Alpha particle. A positively charged particle emitted by some radioactive materials; it consists of two protons and two neutrons and is identical to the nucleus of the helium atom.

Alternating current. A current whose direction of flow periodically reverses itself.

Ammeter. An instrument calibrated to read in amperes the strength of a current flowing in a circuit. For medical purposes, the ampere is too large a unit; hence, it is divided into a thousand parts, or milliamperes. A meter calibrated to read in milliamperes is called a milliammeter.

Ampere. The unit of the rate of transfer of electricity. The international ampere is the unvarying electrical current that, when passed through a solution of silver nitrate in accordance with certain specifications, deposits silver at the rate of 0.001118 g per second.

Amplifier. A device consisting of one or more vacuum tubes, transistors, or magnetic devices and associated components to increase the strength of an applied signal.

Amplitude. The measure of the maximum deviation from zero.

Angstrom. A unit of wavelength of light. It is equal to $\frac{1}{10,000}$ micron or $\frac{1}{10}$ millimicron.

$$\begin{array}{lll}
1 \text{ Angstrom unit} = & .000\ 1 & (\text{or } 10^{-4}) \text{ microns} \\
& .000\ 000\ 1 & (\text{or } 10^{-7}) \text{ millimeters} \\
& .000\ 000\ 01 & (\text{or } 10^{-8}) \text{ centimeters} \\
& .000\ 000\ 000\ 1 & (\text{or } 10^{-10}) \text{ meters}
\end{array}$$

Anelectrotonus. The state of diminished irritability of a nerve or muscle produced in the region near the anode during the passage of an electric current.

Angle of incidence. The angle between a ray incident on a surface and a line drawn perpendicular to the surface at the point of incidence.

Anode. The positive pole of an electrical device. In a thermionic tube, it is sometimes called the plate. When a positive potential is impressed on it from a battery or rectifier, the anode serves as a collector for the electrons emitted from the filament or cathode of the tube.

Arc lamp. Source of light consisting of gaseous particles from the electrodes of an electric arc that are raised to a temperature of incandescence by an electric current.

Atom. The smallest particle of an element. It can exist alone or in combination with like atoms or other elements.

Atomic number. The number of protons in the nucleus of an atom. Each atom has a different atomic number that determines its position in the periodic table.

Atomic weight. The approximate weight of the protons and neutrons in the nucleus of an atom.

Base. The center region of a transistor; that portion of a transistor equivalent to the grid of a vacuum tube.

Bases. Compounds of an alkaline character in solution, capable of reacting with acids to form salts and water; specifically, the hydroxide of a positive element or radical.

Bias. The voltage impressed on the grid of a vacuum tube, relative to the cathode (filament), usually negative.

Bipolar. The use of two poles in electrotherapeutic treatments.

Capacitance. That property of a system of conductors and dielectrics that permits the storage of electric charges.

Capacitor. A device used primarily because it possesses the property of capacitance. It consists of two conducting surfaces separated by a nonconductor or dielectric. A condenser.

Cataphoresis. The transmission of electronegative ions into the body tissues or through a membrane by use of an electric current.

Catelectrotonus. The state of increased excitability produced in a nerve current.

Cathode. The negative pole or electrode of any electrical device. In a thermionic or roentgen-ray tube, it is often identical with the filament; is an emitter of electrons.

Choke coil. A coil having a large inductance, thereby introducing opposition to the flow of alternating current, or choking the current. The higher the frequency of the current that tries to flow, the greater the choking effect. There is no opposition to the flow of direct current.

Chronaxie. Time intensity relation of electric stimuli. The minimal duration for a current pulse having twice the intensity of the rheobasic current.

Circuit breaker. A special switch, arranged to open a circuit quickly and automatically, without injury to itself, when the circuit is overloaded. The usual circuit breaker can be closed or opened by hand, like any switch.

Close coupling. The situation were two circuits or coils are placed in close magnetic proximity to each other, so that the transfer of energy from one to another is large.

Coaxial cable. A two-conductor transmission line in which one conductor completely surrounds the other and acts as a shield for it. An insulating material (dielectric) is placed between the two conductors.

Colloid. A substance that, when apparently dissolved in water or other liquid, diffuses not at all or very slowly through a membrane. Colloids are often gelatinous, like albumen, gelatin, or starch. They generally resemble glue.

Commutator. A device for reversing the direction of an electric current; usually a segmental ring attached to a generator, on which brushes slide.

Condenser. A device for storing up electrical energy. It usually consists of conducting surfaces separated by an insulating medium called the dielectric. A capacitor is a condenser.

Conductance. The property of an electric circuit, or a body used as a part of that circuit, that determines, for a given potential difference between its terminals, the average rate at which electric energy is converted into heat. It is the reciprocal of resistance.

Conductive heat. A term applied to heat transferred by conduction from poultices, bags, etc.

Conductivity. The specific electric conducting ability of a substance.

Constant current. See Direct current.

Continuous current. See Direct current.

Continuous spectrum. An unbroken series of wavelengths, either visible or invisible. Such a spectrum is produced by light from incandescent solids, liquids, or gases under high pressure passed through a prism. Also an unbroken range of radiations of different wavelengths in any portion of the invisible spectrum.

Convective heat. A term used to designate heat that is transferred by convection, as by a stream of air or water.

Conversive heat. A term used to designate heat generated in the tissues by a current of electricity.

Coulomb. The quantity of electricity or the charge transmitted in 1 second by a current of 1 ampere.

Coupling. The amount of flux linkage of one circuit with another. It is a measure of the transfer of energy between two circuits.

Current. The movement of electrons through a conductor. It is measured in amperes.

Cycle. One period of alternating current—that is, the complete sequence of changes from zero to positive maximum, to zero, to negative maximum and back to zero.

Damped current. An oscillating current of electricity in which the amplitude of successive alternations becomes less and less until it finally dies away.

Desiccation. The process of drying up.

Diathermy. The therapeutic use of a high-frequency current to generate heat within some part of the body.

Dielectric. An insulating substance that allows electrostatic induction to act across it, as the insulating medium between the plates of a condenser. An insulating or nonconducting material.

Diode. A two-terminal device that will conduct electricity more easily in one direction than the other.

Direct current. A current that flows in one direction only. When used medically, it is called the "galvanic" current.

Dry heat. In contradistinction to moist heat. Sources of dry heat are the hot water bottle, the electric heating pad, and radiant heat lamps of various types.

Electric circuit. The path through conductors by which an electric current passes.

Electricity. The set of phenomena associated with the existence of electrical charge. See Proton and Electron. It is commonly subdivided into phenomena associated with static charges (electrostatic) and those associated with moving streams of charge (current).

Electrify. To charge a body with electricity.

Electrocautery. An apparatus for cauterizing tissue, consisting of a holder containing a wire that may be heated to a red or a white heat by a current of electricity, either direct or alternating.

Electrocoagulation. Coagulation of tissue by means of a high-frequency electric current. The heat producing the coagulation is generated within the tissue to be destroyed.

Electrocution. The destruction of life by means of electric current.

Electrode. A medium intervening between an electric conductor and the object to which the current is to be applied. In electrotherapy, an electrode is an instrument with a point or a surface from which to discharge current to the body of a patient.

Electrodesiccation. The destructive drying of cells and tissue by means of short high-frequency electric sparks, in contradistinction to fulguration which is the destruction of tissue by means of long high-frequency electric sparks.

Electrodiagnosis. The determination of functional states of various organs and tissues according to their response to electrical stimulation.

Electrolysis. The electrical decomposition of a chemical compound. Examples: the separation of an electrolyte into its constituent parts by a direct current; the removal of hair by the electrolytic effect of a direct current.

Electrolyte. 1. A substance that in solution conducts an electric current and is decomposed by the passage of an electric current. 2. A solution that is a conductor of electricity.

Electromagnetic induction. Generation of an electromotive force in an insulated conductor moving in an electromagnetic field, or in a fixed conductor in a moving magnetic field.

Electromotive force (abbreviation, emf). That effect of difference of potential that, on the closing of a circuit, causes a flow of electricity from one place to another, giving rise to an electric current. The strength of an electric current is directly proportional to the resistance in the case of direct current and to the impedance in the case of alternating current. Electromotive force is measured in volts or in some convenient multiple or fraction of a volt.

Electron. The particle that exists in the outer region of atoms and molecules; it carries the unit negative charge of electricity.

Electronic tube. A vacuum tube evacuated to such a degree that its electrical characteristics are due to electron emission.

Electrophoresis. See Phoresis.

Electrotherapy. Treatment of disease by means of electricity.

Electrothermotherapy. The production of heat within the living tissues for therapeutic purposes by means of bodily resistance to the passing of an electric current.

Electrotonic. Of or pertaining to electrotonus.

Electrotonus. The change in the irritability of a nerve or muscle during the passage of an electric current.

Epilation. Removal of hair.

Erythema. Active hyperemia of the skin indicated by abnormal redness.

Erythema dose. The amount of radiant energy sufficient to evoke perceptible redness of the skin.

Erythemogenic. Causing erythema.

Far ultraviolet radiation. Ultraviolet radiation of short wavelength; farthest away from the visible spectrum.

Farad. A unit of electrical capacity. The capacity of a capacitor that, when charged with 1 coulomb, gives a difference of potential of 1 volt. This unit is so large that one-millionth part of it has been adopted as a practical unit, called a microfarad.

Faradic current. An intermittent, alternating current induced in the secondary winding of an induction coil.

Filament. The cathode of a thermionic tube in which heat is supplied by current passing through it; also the incandescent element in luminous sources of heat.

Filter. A selective circuit network designed to pass currents freely within a continuous band or bands of frequencies, or direct current, and to substantially reduce the amplitude of currents of undesired frequencies. In radiation therapy, screens or various substances that permit passage of some wavelengths while absorbing others.

Fluorescence. Luminescence of a substance when acted on by short-wave light radiation; usually ultraviolet.

Flux. The electromagnetic lines of force, or the magnetic field, produced by a current in a coil.

Fraunhofer's lines. Dark lines of a solar spectrum.

Frequency. The rate of oscillation or alternation in an alternating current circuit, in contradistinction to periodicity in the interruptions or regular variations of current in a direct current circuit. The frequency is computed on the basis of a complete cycle, a complete cycle being one in which the current rises from zero to a maximum, returns to zero, rises to an opposite maximum, and returns to zero again.

Fulguration. See Electrodesiccation.

Full-wave rectifier. A double-element rectifier arranged so the current is allowed to pass in the same direction to the load circuit during each half-cycle of the alternating current supply; one element functions during one half-cycle and the other during next half-cycle.

Fuse. A safety device comprising a strip of wire of easily fusible metal whose conductance is predetermined. The metal fuses and breaks the circuit when an excess of current passes through it.

Galvanic current. A steady unidirectional current.

Galvanism. Therapeutic use of direct current.

Galvanometer. An instrument that measures current by electromagnetic action. It may consist of a magnetic needle delicately suspended in the center of a permanent coil of wire, or a suspended coil between the poles of a fixed magnet. When the current is applied to the coil, the needle is deflected over a calibrated scale. Galvanometers detect current and enable one to determine its direction, amperage, and voltage. The d'Arsonval form is more common, in which a coil moves in a permanent magnetic field. The instrument is called a voltmeter when used in series with a high resistance to measure voltage and an ammeter when used across a shunt to measure amperage.

Gamma rays. Electromagnetic waves that originate in the nucleus of the atom. Gamma rays may have any of a wide range of wavelengths, although the usual gamma ray has a wavelength 10^5 times shorter than visible light wavelengths. X rays come from the electronic structure of the atom and have longer wavelengths.

Grid. An electrode having openings through which electrons or ions may pass. In a thermionic tube, it is generally placed between the cathode and the anode. Its potential controls the current between the cathode and the anode (plate) in a predetermined manner.

Grid voltage. The voltage between a grid and a specified point of the cathode. See also Bias.

Grid voltage supply. The means for supplying and applying with proper regulation the bias or a potential to the grid of a vacuum tube, which is usually negative with respect to the cathode.

Ground. An electrical connection with the earth or with any conductor of large capacity.

Hertz (abbreviation, Hz). Cycles per second.

Hertzian waves. Electromagnetic vibrations that have wavelengths of 1 centimeter or longer.

High frequency. A current having a frequency of interruption or change of direction sufficiently high that tetanic contractions are not set up when it is passed through living contractile tissues.

Hole. In a semiconductor, a mobile vacancy that acts like a positive electronic charge with a positive mass.

Homogeneous. Having the same nature or qualities of uniform character in all parts.

Hot-cathode tube. A vacuum tube in which the cathode is electrically heated (usually to incandescence) in order to increase the emission of electrons.

Hot wire meter. A type of meter used to measure the amperage of high-frequency circuits. The needle of the meter is connected to a wire having a known thermic expansion under the passage of a certain milliamperage, and, as the wire expands, the needle moves across a calibrated scale to indicate the amperage.

Hydroelectric bath. A bath in which electricity is administered to the tissues through water.

Impedance. A measure of the opposition to current flow. It may be caused by resistance, inductance, capacity, or combination of these. The ratio of voltage to current flow in a circuit.

Inductance. The property of an electric circuit by virtue of which a varying current induces an electromotive force in that circuit or in a neighboring circuit

Inductance coil. Wire coiled up so that adjacent turns increase the self-inductance of the wire.

Induction coil. A transformer excited by an interrupted or variable current.

Infrared rays. Radiations just beyond the red end of the spectrum. Their wavelengths range between 770 and 50,000 mμ. The therapeutic range extends from about 770 to 1,400 mμ.

Insulation. The state in which the communication of electricity to other bodies is prevented by the interposition of a nonconductor; also, the material or substance that insulates. The electrical resistance of an insulator is for convenience expressed in megohms, a unit representing a million ohms.

Insulator. A substance or body that interrupts the transmission of electricity to surrounding objects by conduction.

Intensity of electric field. The intensity of an electric field is measured by the force exerted on unit charge. Unit field intensity is the field that exerts the force of one dyne on unit positive charge.

Interrupted current. A current that is frequently opened and closed.

Interrupter. A mechanical or electronic device for making and breaking (closing and opening alternately) an electrical circuit. Such a device is ordinarily employed in low-voltage, direct current circuits.

Inverse square law. The law that states that the intensity of radiation at any distance is inversely proportional to the square of the distance between the irradiated surface and a point source.

Invisible spectrum. Part of the spectrum, either below the red (infrared) or above the violet (ultraviolet), that is invisible to the eye.

Ion. An atom or molecule with a net charge different from zero.

Ionization. The process by which neutral atoms or molecules become charged, either positively or negatively.

Iontophoresis. Synonym of Ion transfer.

Ion transfer. The introduction of chemical ions into the superficial tissues for medicinal purposes by means of a direct current. Iontophoresis.

Irradiation. Application of roentgen rays, radium rays, ultraviolet rays, or other radiation to a patient or object.

Joule. A unit of electrical energy equivalent to work expended when a current of 1 ampere flows for 1 second against a resistance of 1 ohm; a unit of work = 10,000,000 ergs.

Kilocycle. 1000 cycles.

Laser. Acronym for *Light Amplification by Stimulated Emission of Radiation.* A generator and amplifier of coherent energy in the visible or light region of the spectrum.

Leyden jar. A glass jar partially coated, inside and out, with metal, or coated outside with metal and having salt solution inside. It is a capacitor.

Light. The sensation produced by electromagnetic radiation that falls on the retina. Radiant energy producing a sensation of luminosity on the retina, limited to wavelengths from 400 to 700 mμ.

Light therapy. The therapeutic application of radiation in the visible spectrum; some authors include ultraviolet radiation in the term.

Low frequency. An alternating current whose frequency in cycles per second is low. In general, low-frequency currents are attended by tetanic contraction when passed through the body.

Magnetic circuit. The closed path of magnetic lines; e.g., the magnetic circuit of a transformer.

Magnetic field. The space permeated by the magnetic lines of force surrounding a permanent magnet or coil of wire carrying electric current.

Magnetic flux. The total number of lines of induction passing through a surface.

Magnetron. An electron tube that is surrounded by a electromagnet that controls the electron flow from the cathode to the anode.

Mains or main line. The conductors that deliver the current as it comes in from the street supply or from a motor-generator, if one is used.

Megohm. 1,000,000 ohms.

Meter. The unit of length in the metric system; corresponds to 39.37 inches. An instrument or means for measuring some quantity, as a voltmeter.

Mho. The unit of conductivity; the reciprocal of ohm.

Micro. Prefix that means the millionth part. A microampere is the millionth part of an ampere.

Microfarad. $\frac{1}{1,000,000}$ of a farad. A convenient division of the large unit.

Micron. The millionth part of a meter; the thousandth part of a millimeter; 1μ.

Milliammeter. See Ammeter.

Milliampere. One one-thousandth of 1 ampere.

Millimicron. One-millionth of a millimeter; 1 mμ; 10 angstroms; 1 nanometer.

Molecule. A chemical combination of two or more atoms that form a specific chemical substance.

Monochromatic rays. Rays characterized by a definite wavelength.

Motor generator. A device consisting of a motor mechanically connected to a generator. Such machines are designed to generate direct current when alternating alone is available, or *vice versa*.

Nanometer. One millimicron ($m\mu$).

Neutron. An uncharged particle present in all atomic nuclei except the hydrogen nucleus.

Nonconductor. A substance that will not conduct electricity. Strictly speaking, there is no perfect nonconductor. On the application of a sufficiently high voltage, current may be caused to flow through materials usually spoken of as nonconductors. See Insulator.

Ohm. The unit of resistance. The resistance that will allow 1 ampere of current to pass under the pressure due to an electromotive force of 1 volt.

Ohm's law. The law, determined experimentally by the physicist Ohm, that states that the strength of an electric current in a direct current circuit varies directly as the applied electromotive force and inversely as the resistance of the circuit.

Open circuit. A circuit having some break in it so that current is not passing or cannot pass. The break may be intentional, as an open switch, or accidental, as a blown fuse, a loose connection, or a broken wire.

Oscillating current. A current alternating in direction, and of either constant or gradually decreasing amplitude. An oscillating current of constant amplitude is called an undamped current; one of gradually increasing amplitude, a damped current.

Oscillatory circuit. One that offers very little opposition to the establishment of an oscillating current of the frequency to which it is tuned.

Oscilloscope. An instrument for making visible the nature and form of oscillations or irregularities of an electric current.

Oudin current. A high-frequency current of higher voltage than the high-frequency currents used for long-wave diathermy treatments (obsolete).

Parallel connection. One in which the current divides and passes along more than one path.

Period. In an alternating current, the time required for one cycle to pass through a complete set of positive and negative values.

Periodicity. The rate of interruption of a unidirectional electric current.

Phoresis. The migration of ions through a membrane by the action of an electric current.

Phosphorescence. The induced luminescence that persists after cessation of the irradiation that caused it.

Photoluminescence. The light emission of an object that becomes luminescent when acted on by light.

Photometer. A device for measuring the intensity of light.

Photosynthesis. A chemical combination caused by the action of light.

Phototaxis. The movement of cells and microorganisms under the influence of light.

Physiatrics. The science that relates to the medicinal and curative application of physical forces, such as light, heat, and electricity.

Physiatrist. The physician who practices physiatrics.

Physical therapist. A medical graduate skilled in physical therapy.

Physical therapy. Physical therapy is the therapeutic use of physical agents. It comprises the use of physical, chemical, and other properties of heat, light, water, electricity, massage, and exercise. See also **Physiatrics**.

Piezoelectric. The property exhibited by some crystals that causes a voltage to be produced when it is subjected to a mechanical stress and, conversely, a mechanical stress to be produced when it is subjected to a voltage.

Plate. The positively charged platelike element in a vacuum tube that collects the electrons emitted by the filament or cathode. A term commonly used for the anode.

Plate circuit. All the devices connected directly in the external circuit between the filament and the plate elements.

Polarity. 1. The fact or condition of having poles. 2. The exhibition of opposite effects at the two extremities.

Positive rays. Streams of positively charged atoms traveling at high speed from the anode of a partially evacuated tube under the influence of an applied voltage.

Potential. A condition by which current tends to flow from a place of higher to one of lower potential. The practical unit of measurement is the volt.

Potentiometer. An arrangement for securing any desired voltage by utilizing the voltage drop across a portion of current-carrying resistance.

Power. Rate at which work is being done. The electrical unit of power is the watt. See Watt.

Preamplifier. An amplifier that raises the output of a low-level source so that it may be further amplified by a later stage. A preamplifier often includes provisions for equalization and mixing.

Proton. The nucleus of the hydrogen atom. It carries the unit positive charge of electricity. See Electron.

Pulsating current. A current pulsating regularly in magnitude. As ordinarily used, applies to a unidirectional current.

Quantum. As much as; a certain specified quantity or amount; an elementary unit of energy; the supposed atom of light.

Quartz. Silicon dioxide, the principal ingredient of sandstone (crystallized silica; rock crystals). When crystal is clear and colorless, it permits the passage of ultraviolet radiations in large proportions. Also used to change high-frequency current to ultrasound vibrations.

Quartz glass. Crystalline quartz is used for prisms and lenses, fused quartz for windows, etc., through which ultraviolet radiations are freely transmitted.

Radar. An acronym for *Radio Detection and Ranging.* A system for measuring the distance (and usually direction) to an object by measuring the time required for a signal to travel to the object and return.

Radiant energy. That form of energy that is transmitted through space without the support of a sensible medium. Radio waves, infrared rays, visible rays, ultraviolet rays, roentgen rays, gamma rays, and cosmic rays are energy in this form.

Radiation. A general term for any form of radiant energy, emission, or divergence, as of energy in all directions from luminous bodies, roentgen-ray tubes, radioactive elements, fluorescent substances, or from an antenna.

Radio frequency. Current of frequency above 10,000 cycles per second; currents of this frequency and higher are easily radiated by an antenna.

Radiotherapy. The treatment of disease by application of roentgen rays, radium, and other radiations.

Rationale. A rational exposition of principles; the logical basis of a procedure.

Reactance. That component of impedance or opposition to flow of accelerating current produced by capacitance or inductance. The ratio between the voltage and that component of the current that is 90 degrees out of phase with the voltage.

Rectifier. A device that converts alternating current into unidirectional current by permitting appreciable flow of current in one direction only.

Refraction. The change of direction of a ray when it passes from one medium to another of a different optical density.

Relay. A device by which contacts in one circuit are operated by a change in conditions in the same circuit or in one or more associated circuits.

Resistance. The opposing influence of a body (solid, liquid, or gaseous) to the passage of an electric current. It is expressed in ohms; 1 ohm allows 1 ampere of current to flow at a pressure of 1 volt. The effect of the expenditure of electrical energy in resistance is to generate heat.

Resonance. Two circuits are in resonance if they are in tune with each other—that is, if the products of the inductance and capacity of each are equal.

Resonator. An electrical circuit in which oscillations of a certain frequency are set up by oscillations of the same frequency in another circuit. When this occurs, the circuits are said to be in syntony.

Rheobase. The voltage required for a minimal response with the make of the current in electric stimulation.

Rheostat. A fixed or variable resistance for controlling the amount of current entering a circuit.

Ripple current. A pulsating current, superimposed on a direct current. The constant component is usually large relative to the sum of the amplitudes of the harmonic components.

Roentgen rays. Radiation associated with the sudden change in velocity of free electrons (general radiation) or the transfer from higher to lower energy levels of electrons bound in atoms (characteristic radiation). "Roentgen rays" is preferred by medical authorities, but "x rays" is in more general use by physicians. The wavelengths concerned are usually between 0.005 and 1 millimicron.

Roentgen-ray tube. A glass vacuum bulb containing two electrodes. Electrons are obtained either from gas in the tube or from a heated cathode. When suitable potential is applied, electrons travel at high velocity from cathode to anode, where they are suddenly arrested, giving rise to roentgen rays.

Screens. See Filters.

Secondary. In a transformer, the output winding.

Self-inductance. The property of an electric circuit that determines, for a given rate of change of current in the circuit, the electromotive force induced in the circuit itself.

Semiconductor. A material that has electrical conductivity between that of a conductor and that of an insulator: a device made from such material.

Series. A mode of arranging the parts of a circuit by connecting them successively end to end to form a single path for the current. The parts so arranged are said to be "in series."

Short circuit. An accidental overflow of current due to the establishment of a low-resistance bypass.

Shunt. When two or more electrical devices or resistances are so connected that the current is divided between them, the current through each device or resistance being inversely proportioned to the resistance, they are said to be connected "in shunt" or in parallel with one another.

Sinusoidal current. Also see Alternating current. An alternating current following in the sine law.

Solarium. A room designed for heliotherapy or for the application of artificial light.

Solenoid. A coil or series of turns of wire spaced equally between turns. Usually designates a coil whose length is greater than its diameter. When an electric current flows through a solenoid, the solenoid acts in general like a magnet.

Spark gaps. Arrangement of opposed points or surfaces between which an electric spark may jump.

Spectrograph. An instrument designed to photograph spectra on a sensitive photographic plate.

Spectrometer. A spectroscope so constructed that the angular deviation of a ray of light produced by a prism or by a diffraction grating, thus indicating the wavelength of the light, can be accurately measured.

Spectroscope. An instrument for separating radiant energy into its component frequencies or wavelengths by means of a prism or grating.

Spectroscopy. The branch of physical science that treats of the phenomena observed with the spectroscope, or those principles on which its action is based; also, the art of using the spectroscope.

Spectrum. Charted band of wavelengths of electromagnetic vibrations obtained by refraction or diffraction. The visible spectrum consists of the colors from red to violet. The invisible spectrum is composed of Hertzian rays, infrared rays, ultraviolet rays, roentgen rays (x rays), gamma rays, and cosmic rays.

Static electricity. Electricity produced by friction.

Step-down transformer. A transformer in which the number of turns of wire in the primary and secondary windings is such as to reduce voltage. (See Transformer.)

Step-up transformer. A transformer in which the number of turns of wire in the primary and secondary windings is such as to increase voltage. (See Transformer.)

Surgical diathermy. The use of high-frequency electrical oscillations in such a way that animal tissues are destroyed.

Tension. Sometimes used as a synonym for voltage; thus high tension would mean high voltage.

Thermal. Pertaining to heat. Thermal unit = the amount of heat required to raise the temperature of a given mass of water by $1°$ F or C. Common thermal units are the Btu, the heat required to raise 1 pound of water $1°$ F, and the Calorie, the amount of heat required to raise 1 gram of water $1°$ C. Thermal capacity: the amount of heat required to raise temperature of a body from $0°$ to $1°$ C.

Thermionic rectifier. A device that converts alternating current into direct current. It is an electric valve in which the electrons are supplied by a heated electrode.

Thermionic tube. A tube in which the electron emission is produced by the heating of an electrode.

Thermoelectric effect. The voltage effect generated at the terminals of a junction of two dissimilar metals; it is greater with some metals than with others.

Thermopile. A thermoelectric battery used in measuring small variations in the degree of heat. It consists of a number of dissimilar metallic plates connected together, in which, under the influence of heat, an electric current is produced.

Thermotherapy. The therapeutic application of heat.

Tickler. A coil in the plate circuit used to feed some of the energy back into the grid circuit.

Transformer. A device used for transferring electrical energy from one circuit to another, usually by magnetic-field effect.

Transistor. A semiconductor device analogous in action to a vacuum tube that has at least three leads.

Tuned circuit. A circuit is said to be tuned when its natural period of oscillation is the same as that of some other circuit to which it is coupled.

Tuning. The operation of adjusting any circuit to be in electrical resonance with any other circuit or circuits.

Ultrasound. High-frequency (about 1 million per sec) vibrations or sound waves.

Ultraviolet radiation. Radiation characterized by invisible rays in the electromagnetic spectrum between the violet rays and the roentgen rays. In wavelength, it ranges from 400 to 20 mμ. It possesses powerful actinic and chemical properties.

Undamped current. An alternating current of electricity in which the amplitude of successive alternations is maintained.

Unidirectional. The state of transmission in one direction, as electric currents in a circuit.

Vacuum tube. A vessel of insulating material (usually glass) provided with metal electrodes that has been so highly evacuated that the residual gas does not affect the current between the electrodes.

Variable condenser. One whose electrical capacity may be changed or varied.

Variometer. Two coils that may be placed in such relative positions that the inductance effects of each winding may be made to assist or practically neutralize each other.

Volt. The unit of electromotive force. The electrical pressure required to send a current of 1 ampere through the resistance of 1 ohm.

Voltage. Electromotive force or difference in potential expressed in volts.

Voltmeter. A meter designed and calibrated to measure voltage. Voltmeters are connected in parallel with the circuit or resistance over which the potential drop is to be measured.

Water-cooled quartz mercury vapor arc lamp. A small quartz mercury vapor arc lamp enclosed in a double-walled metal box with a quartz window for generation and application of ultraviolet rays. Water is circulated between the walls to conduct away the intense heat. Often called a Kromayer lamp after the inventor, Dr. E. Kromayer.

Watt. The unit of electrical power. The product of current and electromotive force.

Wattage. The power output or consumption of an electrical device expressed in watts.

Watt-hour. An electrical unit of work of energy. It is equal to the wattage multiplied by the time in hours. Its mechanical equivalent is 2,655 foot-pounds.

Watt meter. A meter for measuring electric power.

Wave. A single impulse, or the disturbance included in a space of one wavelength, or the advance of a disturbance into a medium.

Wavelength.   The distance between corresponding points in two adjacent waves; e.g., between two crests. In therapeutic radiations, it is stated in angstroms or in millimicrons. The term "angstroms" is becoming obsolete.

Wave meter.   A measuring device, arranged and calibrated to read the length of a radiated wave directly in meters.

Wave train.   A series of waves, of the same or diminishing amplitude, usually repeating after intervals of inaction.

Wood's filter.   A screen that absorbs visible rays but allows a portion of the ultraviolet rays to be transmitted.

X rays.   See Roentgen rays.

Index

Page numbers in italic indicate figures; page numbers followed by t indicate tables.

261